GUARDIANS OF THE FRONTLINE

Randy J Hopper, RRT

1

FIRST PRINTING EDITION MMXX

Contents

Disclaimer

During the Covid-19 pandemic, I was a frontline worker in New York City and other hotspots. As a travelling Respiratory Therapist, I went into some of hottest of the hot spots during the pandemic and garnered a lot of memorable experiences that I want to share.

This story is based upon facts as I understood them on the ground. I have taken every attempt not to politicize the virus and be as accurate as possible.

However, certain names and instances were altered to protect the innocent. It isn't my intention to harm anyone. I merely want to tell the story of Covid-19 from the frontline perspective and share my experiences with anyone who's willing to listen.

Be advised that I am not a medical doctor – but I am a medical professional. We are the guardians of the frontline. And any opinions expressed herein are mine and mine alone.

I have taken every effort to tell this story as accurately as possible – with the best scientific information available to me at the time I wrote this book – but I cannot guarantee the accuracy of anything discussed as things are rapidly evolving.

Keep in mind: this is not about politics. It's about saving lives – and figuring out the best ways to do that using the best information available to us at the time.

Acknowledgements

Who are the guardians of the frontline? They are people you know and some people you may not know but have read about. They look like me and you. They come in all shapes, colors, sizes, and backgrounds. They have taken an oath to help you and people you love. They have willingly gone into the frontlines of this pandemic while risking their own lives to provide care for people they will never know. For those reasons, I wanted to give a special thank you to all my colleagues on the frontlines who are continuing to do a great job to this day. We have lost a lot of people in this battle, but there's no telling how many more people we would have lost if not for their work.

Forward

What started out like a small spark in the forest quickly turned into a raging wildfire. The virus, which had seemingly appeared out of nowhere, was now all over the place. And no one was sure how the outbreak occurred. Of course, there have been many theories, ranging from improbable to somewhat logical to outright absurd and counterproductive. It is incredible what can be passed as true if you are spoon-fed enough of it.

Some people postulated that the virus started with a bat-eating lunatic on a feeding frenzy somewhere in China. Others said it was caused by new 5G networks in Wuhan. They argued that 5G was a means to spread the virus. Others said the virus was a trojan horse tucked away inside the flu vaccine, and that it was an intentional act aimed at turning all of us into mindless zombies.

The theories ran amok, and it was all enough to make your head spin. I guess the most believable story I heard was that the coronavirus was the result of an unfortunate series of events that started in earnest in a research laboratory in China. Researchers were experimenting with a new strand of SARS when the virus somehow slipped out into the public sphere.

You know, I don't think anyone knows for sure how the virus started. And I'm no longer concerned with such details in any case. I'm far more concerned with the havoc the virus is recking on the global community.

Not to mention, there is one indisputable fact that I have come to understand: the coronavirus does not discriminate.

People all over the world have been infected and died. People are continuing to be affected as of the time of the writing of this book. The Grim Reaper has been putting in lots of overtime as I struggle to write these words.

It's a nasty little virus. That much is certain. And it's incredibly efficient at doing one thing rather well: killing. It is silent, but it is brutal. It attacks the respiratory system with a vengeance, and the results of which are a weakened immune system, failing organs, and death.

As a Respiratory Care Practitioner, I understand these facts better than most, and I have seen the results of the virus to the body up close and personal. In short, I had the great privilege of being a guardian on the frontline, an experience that I will likely never forget. I worked alongside exceptional Respiratory Therapist and other healthcare professionals. You see, the memories of what the virus does to its victims are forever etched into my memory, and so I recently decided to share my experiences with the world.

The human body is incredibly clever and all connected. One system cannot work correctly unless the other systems are working correctly.

In fact, if the human body were a caboose, the lungs would be the coal-burning part of the train that kept it running. Oxygen must pass through the lungs to feed the tissues to keep the body going. If you stop that process in any way, you are bound to have some significant issues. And by issues, I mean death, which is what is happening so devastatingly well with this virus, a form of SARS.

The virus comes in many names, SARS-Cov2, Covid-19, and the coronavirus chief amongst them. There are even some less sensitive names that I will choose to ignore.

When it burst onto the scene in late-2019, I was like many of you, I imagine. I assumed it would be quarantined to China – and that most of the rest of the world had truly little to worry about. Boy was I wrong.

My anxieties would quickly grow as I watched the virus spread to other countries. I feared that if not stopped it would reach our shores – and it was getting more and more likely that was going to happen.

In the beginning, we were assured that it would be contained. Many of our elected officials mindlessly repeated, "We have nothing to worry about!"

But we now know how badly wrong they played their hand. Things continued to get worse – and, in many ways, they still are.

The curve is not flattened outside of one or two places like New Zealand. People are still dying left and right. Morgues have been overflowing in hotspots throughout the world. Medical professionals are putting in long hours and becoming increasingly exhausted at the sheer workload and the horrendous nature of what they are witnessing. Some of them are even quitting or retiring early due to the toll of the job.

In all fairness, the virus spread much faster than many of us anticipated, at least at first. Wearing masks in public has become the new normal. Quarantining in your home is was a new normal, too. And people are separated from their family and friends in ways we cannot imagine.

I look at quarantining like a test of wills. Human beings thrive on the connections they make and manage. Without all those intimate connections, there are tons of psychological effects on the mind and body. Isolation leads to restlessness and pinned-up energy that cannot be properly vented. Even introverts occasionally crawl out of their holes to connect with others.

Coverage of the virus is nonstop. It's pretty much all you hear about whether that's on social media or television or beyond. Vaccine and antibody trials have started throughout the world. And a race against time has ensued to get the virus under control, relieve the pressure on our healthcare infrastructure, and, hopefully, if we do things exactly right, save as many lives as possible.

So, what is the result from a societal standpoint? Well, much of it you have experienced yourself, and I will not reiterate here. But suffice it to say, many people are turning against one another in droves. The political climate is at a new high. Divisiveness is rampant.

We've somehow managed to politicize a stinking virus!

God forbid you have a cough or happen to sneeze in public. People will assume you have the zombie plague and will avoid you like the plague.

Going out is not the same. Restaurants were closed for some time – and only just recently have many of them been allowed to reopen with restrictions. Tables are starting to spill over into sidewalks and streets.

Social distancing has forced the world to find creative ways to bring people together safely. Gatherings have become these awkward "together but separate at the same time" events where people are still trying to cope with the new reality.

It's not the same. 2020 is a watershed moment in recent human history. That much is true, and what the world looks like coming out of this year is still unclear.

I have never seen anything like it. I'm not sure anyone has – unless you lived through the Spanish Flu, but things were much different back then, so I don't think there's really any comparison that would make sense. In short, these are unchartered waters if I might borrow the cliché.

I feel like the world has catapaulted into a new level of pandemonium, which we see manifest everywhere we turn. People are more fearful than ever, yet they still strive for those social connections that they once thrived on and yearned for.

Of course, I know that we will get through this, but at what cost? In what ways have you already been affected? How did we get into this situation? Where are we heading? And what lessons can be learned?

These are just a few of the lingering concerns that many of you probably already have contemplated.

I feel comfortable saying that we will adapt, persevere, and ultimately, overcome. Someday the virus will be a fading memory of a chaotic time period. Hopefully, we will have learned some valuable lessons along the way that will help us prevent the next big pandemic.

The coronavirus will be a footnote in history, and more stories like this one will pop up, reminding us of the cost we paid (some more dearly than others).

In fact, I am reminded of some of my own experiences with the virus, especially my days working the frontlines. As a travelling Respiratory Therapist, I was on the ground in some of the worst hotspots in the country.

The memories I made and the experiences I shared will last a lifetime. And currently, I'd like to share some of those experiences with you. I don't recall the exact day when this story begins, but let's flashback to early March 2020.

Chapter 1

The Bachelor's Dream

I t was a cool, overcast morning in March when my alarm clock rang, reminding me it was six o'clock. I slung my arm at the end table as the clock crashed to the floor and bounced. My head was a little bit groggy, and I just laid there for a bit longer collecting my thoughts.

To be honest, I dreaded rolling those warm, comfy blankets back. I felt so comfortable bundled up in my bed and briefly contemplated calling into work.

Before long it hit me.

What the hell are you doing? I wondered.

I never miss work. Hell, I love work. I live for the excitement of being in the emergency room. I enjoy helping others and knowing what I do makes a difference in people's lives (sometimes the difference between life and death).

It was time to start my day whether I was ready or not, so I coaxed myself up and out of bed and finally silenced the alarm that was practically bouncing across my bedroom floor at that point.

The whole apartment was cool and dark. The sun had yet to stir – or it was tucked behind some clouds hiding. And with the recent changes in the weather, it was a constant battle to get the thermostat to the perfect setting. Dial it up one small increment, and before you know it, you're burning up. Turn it down ever so slightly, and you'll be grabbing a blanket or hoody in no time.

I elected for a heavier pajama top and quickly slipped it over my head and then headed for the kitchen to make myself a bowl of cereal.

Hey, don't judge me! I'm actually a surprisingly good cook, but who's got time for that? Cooking is more of an extravagance these days – and I'm still living the bachelor's "dream."

After settling for some Captain Crunch, which is all I had left in my pantry, I filled the bowl to the brim with almond milk, grabbed a spoon from the drawer, and made my way to the living room.

The TV was still on from the previous night but was turned all the way down as some familiar-looking talking head flapped his gums to no sound. I started pushing buttons on the remote control, and soon, the entire room filled up with noise.

I fell into my oversized sofa and started scarfing down the tasty morsels as the network anchor explained all the recent news related to Covid-19. In recent weeks, the virus had escaped from China and was now raging in Italy and other countries. Images of overrun hospitals and body bags filled the screen as I gasped in horror.

They had these reefer trucks pulled up at a hospital there, which were apparently used for overflows from the hospital morgues. Let me tell you: in all my experience, that isn't normal. People just don't ordinarily die at those rates to justify something like that.

If it can do all of that damage and destruction over there, I thought, there's no reason why it can't happen here.

I continued to listen as they brought in an expert who tried to describe the situation in Washington state, which was intensifying in recent days. There were only a handful of cases tied to a cruise ship at the time, but I still couldn't shake the images of Italy from before.

I don't recall his name – and it's not really all that important – but it was clear that he wasn't worried about the coronavirus recking havoc in the United States like it was doing in Italy. He was acting like everything was under control.

He then quoted the mayor of New York who had apparently encouraged New Yorkers to go on with their lives and get out on the town despite the coronavirus. I couldn't help but think how odd those words seemed, especially in hindsight.

Are they serious? I thought.

I looked at what's happening in Italy – and then I thought about the basic mood of everyone in the U.S. at the time. Most people were completely oblivious to just how bad this virus was, and to be clear, even as a medical professional, I was somewhat unclear myself.

I also had this foreboding feeling in the pit of my stomach that something wasn't right. I felt like things were doomed to get worse here. I felt like it was more of a matter of time.

That is to say, it wasn't if the virus would spread throughout America, it was when.

After finishing off my bowl of cereal I added it to my collection of dirty dishes in the sink before heading for the bathroom to get ready for my day.

The only problem was I couldn't quite shake those images of all the dead bodies in reefer trucks – and all the madness in those Italian ER's – from my memory. I felt terrible for them – and hoped beyond hope that we would never experience that kind of pain and suffering here.

I guess you could say I had confidence in our healthcare infrastructure. As a frontline employee, I see firsthand how well our healthcare is compared to many other places. But I also knew not to take this virus lightly, and my fear at that time was that was exactly what was happening.

Worse than that, we were somehow politicizing the Covid-19 pandemic, a point that's still bugged me to this day.

. . .

Every day at work I talked with doctors and other medical professionals about the virus. I was starting to get a clearer picture for what we were dealing with – but there were a lot of unknown variables, and that troubled me to no end.

Recall what I said about the governor? I don't mean to single him out, by the way. People from both sides of the aisle were not taking this virus seriously at first. But suffice it to say, within a few short weeks, people were no longer being told to go out on the town and act like nothing was happening. It was becoming way too much to ignore.

Plus, the RT's and other staff at my work were concerned, and if I've learned one thing in my career in the medical industry, it's that when Respiratory gets concerned, you should too.

I guess that makes sense, right?

It's not like they could take the virus lightly with so many cases popping up every day lately.

Think of it like this: in early March, there was only a few cases per day in the New York City for comparison. But by the first of April they were seeing an average rate of new cases of over 7,000 per day. Imagine that

With a population of almost 9 million people in that city and an estimated R-0 of about 2.5 (if not higher), there was no doubt the entire city would be completely inundated in no time.

I found myself watching the news more and more in those days, which is not something that I was accustomed to doing.

It's like all my anxieties were coming to the surface, and the news wasn't helping things much. They had gone from cognitive dissonance or entirely indifferent to an oh-my-God-the-sky-is-falling mentality in a few short weeks.

Cable news was the worst. There were more twists and turns than a slummy soap opera, and it was impossible to keep up.

I had also just found out about travelling Respiratory Therapists (RT's) jobs, which is an idea that intrigued me a great deal. I couldn't hardly set back any longer while the virus raged on and on and do nothing about it.

So, I picked up my cellphone and called one of my colleagues who got me in touch with a travelling agency.

From there, things started moving briskly. I was going to trade in my bachelor's dream for a position on the frontlines.

Chapter 2

Seeds of Doubt

Flash forward a few months and I was already working for the travel agency in temporary spots throughout the country for a little while. But the whole time, I felt completely unsatisfied. Every day I would get home and find out the new case and death counts in New York City, and wish I could be there helping.

That's right about when I picked up my phone and called my recruiter.

"Book me on the first flight to New York," I proudly proclaimed.

"Wow, wow, wow," he said. "Slow down. You're supposed to be going to Seattle next, and they need help, too."

"Have you seen what's going on in New York?"

"Of course, I have. It's all over the news. And to be fair, I got some contacts there, but there's no way I can get you into New York right now. Too much red tape. I'm sorry. I really need you in Seattle."

I hesitated for a second and then agreed. Who was I to argue? I thought.

I was making good money travelling, doing what I loved, and helping people in the process. So, it was settled then. As it turns out, it didn't appear like there was enough time to go to New York anyway. To be honest, I didn't sign up for my license in time to leave, so the decision was basically made for me.

I couldn't blame him or anyone else. I've always had a big problem with procrastination. Just writing this book was an event itself. I'm so busy working all the time, it was hard to find the time and discipline myself and to get it done.

I stared at the television screen as the numbers for New York City continued to flash across.

My heart ached for the people there.

"Okay," I said, relenting. "Seattle it is."

"Are you ready to leave?"

"I can be."

"Well, let's make it happen," he declared.

"How fast can you get me there?"

"How fast can you pack?"

"That quickly, huh?"

"Yes sir."

After the call, I looked around my little apartment and did a quick accounting of my life up until that point.

I had a nice job. I was already helping people. I made decent money. Everything was going well. Sure, it would be exciting to go to New York, but it wasn't going to happen, so I would have to suck it up and go where they sent me.

For some context, our agency was sending Respiratory Therapists, which is what I am, and other medical professionals to various hospitals in need of extra man (and woman) power during the crisis. New York, Seattle, Massachusetts, Rhode Island. *Shout out to my Rhode Islanders.* These were just a few of the places that needed us the most, but each state and locality had its own requirements that must be met before going there.

In my case, I wanted to go to New York, but they had some rigorous requirements to get started to put it mildly.

After that convo, the whole thing happened quickly, too.

The entire process took maybe two, three days at the most to complete, and I was ready to head out.

My flight was booked. My rental car was secured. I was all packed up, had my affairs in order. I was going to hop on the next plane bound for Seattle for the seven-hour trek across the country.

I'm not sure if it was divine intervention or something less dubious – but sitting around watching the madness on TV was no longer good enough for me. Sometimes you must roll your sleeves back and get your hands a little bit dirty; at least, that's what my grandfather always taught me, and I think he was right.

. . .

The next day I was on my way to the airport. Like I said, it all happened extremely fast, but I needed a change of direction. My hands were sweating. I do that when I get nervous.

I was already having some second thoughts as I scrolled my phone and researched the latest numbers, something I had gotten very accustomed to doing lately.

"Where you flying to?" the Uber driver asked, turning onto the main highway. Pretty soon my little apartment was a speck in the rearview mirror as he pressed the accelerator down harder, and we propelled down the highway.

"Seattle," I said. My adventure had officially begun.

"That right?"

"Well, that's what they tell me, bro."

"They?" he asked, quizzically.

I grinned and then bit my tongue. Sometimes less words are best.

I stared back into my phone. My heart was still in New York – but it was increasingly clear I wasn't going there. So, I looked up the numbers for Washington this time.

Let's see what's going on, I thought, scrolling with my finger down the screen.

Apparently, since the first confirmed cases of the coronavirus in King County, life in the region was virtually upended as state and local officials tried to slow the spread of the virus.

Throughout the month of March, officials passed down a series of orders that surprised most people, but I knew what they were trying to do.

With so many unknowns at that time, they were just trying to slow spread and minimize the effects on the healthcare infrastructure.

The spread of the virus was impacting practically every aspect of life, especially there (and elsewhere). If you recall, Washington was the first hotspot in the United States.

I kept scrolling through my phone, reading the data and various news reports were coming out of the region.

Residents were trying to settle into what has become a new normal, one article said, and they were following social distancing guidelines and staying at home as much as possible.

It's unclear exactly how long these social distancing orders will need to stay in place, but officials recently said that what people are doing appears to be working to slow the spread of the virus.

The first known death in that state – and the entire country as it occurred – due to the novel coronavirus was reported on February 29 to be exact.

On that same day, the governor of that state, Gov. Inslee, announced a state of emergency due to the virus, saying it would allow officials there to get the resources needed to continue to fight the virus.

One of the resources he was referring to were ventilators, which, as it occurs, is part of my job description.

As an RT, I'm the guy who manages the ventilator, should you need to be placed on one. I make sure that it's done properly, and everything works and continues to work safely.

A ventilator is the last-ditch effort to save someone's life when they have this virus, and, at the time, they were in high demand as you can imagine.

In the first week of March, companies in the area were urging employees to work from home. From the beginning of the month, a lot of companies had encouraged any employees who could work remotely to do so, including some of the biggest employers in the country, Amazon, Microsoft, and many others.

I paused from my reader and thought about all the small business that had been impacted, too.

Think about all those little arts and crafts boutiques, mom and pop bars and restaurants. They were all effected, some worse than others. Some would close – and never reopen. So, it was something that the larger corporations could handle better for obvious reasons.

Plus, around that same time, the schools were also starting to close down, too. Some of them had closed down for cleanings after someone experienced symptoms or was in contact with someone who had tested positive.

Other schools had closed for training in the event they did get shut down for an extended period, which, in hindsight, certainly makes sense.

On March 3, the Seattle mayor issued his own proclamation of civil emergency. The order gave Mayor Jenny Durkan the ability to exercise executive power to address immediate dangers to the public, in her words.

The Uber driver said something else – but I was completely locked into reading. I get that way sometimes. And I wasn't about to step off that plane without knowing what the hell I was getting myself into.

So, King County, which is the county where Seattle resides, had already announced plans to buy a motel to use as a quarantine site.

On March 6, the number of confirmed cases of Covid, to put this into perspective, across the state had topped 100, which, to many people, still seemed like extraordinarily little.

And then on the 11th of that month, the governor banned gatherings of 250 people or more in certain counties, including where I was heading. The order came as several events had already started to be canceled or postponed because of the spread of the virus.

Within a week, he had expanded that ban to the entire state of Washington as the virus began to spread more rapidly than before.

On the 13th, Seattle closed all community centers and public libraries, as well as pools and other recreational facilities.

At that same time, Gov. Inslee announced all schools across the state would have to close for at least six weeks. Specifically, his announcement meant that all K-12 public and private schools must close their doors by March 17. At first, that proclamation would last through the end of April.

On March 13, the city of Seattle issued a moratorium on residential evictions for the nonpayment of rent, which made sense because thousands of people had been effectively laid off due to the virus.

On the 16th, the number of confirmed cases across the state topped 1,000 for the first time, and anyone who was thinking the virus would be stopped before it continued to spread were now in the minority, anecdotally speaking.

Think about it. They had 100 cases ten days previously. Now they had over 1,000 by that point, so the infection rate (commonly called the R-0 in academic circles) was not something to be taken lightly.

On March 16, all restaurants, bars, gyms, and entertainment facilities were officially closed, but they still made exceptions for takeout and delivery, which I felt like was a good thing since I would be eating out a lot most likely.

The state did other things too, like extending the moratorium on evictions to the whole state. The governor also waved the one-week waiting period for unemployment, as it became abundantly clear that the coronavirus was here to stay, at least for the foreseeable future.

Doubt crept in my mind.

Was I making the right decision? I wondered.

By March 22, King County alone topped the 1,000 mark for confirmed cases, including 106 new cases on that day. A new death was also reported, bringing the total of confirmed deaths in that county to 75.

Flashforward a little bit longer, on April 5, new guidelines for people to start wearing face masks in public were finally recommended.

And around that same time, it was announced the governor had donated 400 ventilators from the national stockpile to other places that needed them like New York, which was continuing to struggle to get enough equipment to fight the increasing number of cases.

Finally, on April 6, he announced that schools would be closed for the rest of the academic year, and students in those schools would continue to use the distance learning model they had already been using.

I kept scrolling my phone as my anxiety kept increasing more and more. I thought about what it must be like to be in a hotspot versus just reading about it on my phone or hear about these places on TV.

Pretty soon, all the horrific headlines I had read would be my new reality.

Italy came to mind, too.

Oh my God, I thought.

I knew we couldn't go down the same track Italy had taken in the early days of the virus. First, I figured, we had to recognize the seriousness of the situation.

At that time, it was still pretty common to see both citizens and government officials who were skeptical about Covid-19, pointing to low fatality rates, and asking why there was such a panic, given how many folks die of the flu each year.

That was one of the biggest problems I saw. This isn't the flu. It's novel. It spreads stealth-like. Some people who spread it aren't even showing any symptoms for days.

The gravity of their illness may not become clear until a week or two or after being infected if ever. In hindsight, maybe these were the seeds of doubt that had been planted for the explosion in the United States to happen.

Italian leaders did not act preemptively despite evidence that seemed to suggest that such delays would increase cases. Emergency declarations were simply shrugged off by the citizens and the political leaders.

On my way to the airport I was reminded of those same lax attitudes I saw all around, reflecting the same confirmation bias in the United States and elsewhere.

The first thing we should have done was to acknowledge the current situation for what it was – but who am I to preach?

It's just that seeing politicians, who I will not name, totally downplay the virus as a real threat was starting to bug me a little bit if I were being honest. Mixed messages were sent. And after finally being forced to take more stringent measures, the virus was already spreading.

There was this whole selective approach that may have very well inadvertently facilitated the spread of Covid-19. It was all very infuriating.

I was still looking down at my phone when we pulled up at the airport. I didn't even notice that we had come to a complete stop.

"Ready?" he said.

"Sorry?" I replied, looking up.

"We're here."

"Oh, I'm sorry."

I grabbed the door handle and paused briefly.

Maybe the driver could anticipate my seeds of doubt when he shot me a "Good luck."

I pulled the handle and stepped outside. He met me at the back of the vehicle to help me with my bags, and we exchanged a few final cordialities.

Finally, I placed my phone on airplane mode, tucked it into my pocket, and grabbed my luggage from his outstretched hands.

I made a vow to keep my phone in my pocket for a few hours. I guess I was drowning in some terrible combination of headlines, data, and anxiety.

What the hell am I getting myself into? I wondered, as I strolled inside.

Chapter 3

Divine Intervention

Remember when I said something about divine intervention earlier? I'm not sure if you believe in that sort of thing. I do. Let me elaborate.

One of the first things I noticed when I entered the airport was the lack of people.

Well, it wasn't completely empty or anything like that. But things were certainly different. If you've ever been to an airport, and I've been to plenty, they are usually hopping with passengers from all around the world, pilots, staff, and others, hurrying off in all directions.

They are alive with energy. Hugs all around. People laughing. People crying. Energy.

Not this one.

For one, it was about one-third as busy as normal, I would guestimate, which is kind of nice, I suppose, because I didn't have to wait in line very long to get screened.

I laid my computer case and the small carry-on bag I was holding on the counter. I showed the TSA guard my ID who shot it a quick look and then handed it back.

He asked for my ticket, and I scrambled for my phone and pulled it up online. I hardly ever use physical tickets anymore. Gotta love technology.

Satisfied I wasn't a threat he finally said, "Right this way." He motioned me into a huge metal detector.

I sat my phone, wallet, and keys in the plastic bin and stepped inside the huge machine with my arms and hands stretched out in every direction as it detected my every orifice for metal.

After the scan, I grabbed my belongings, and I was off to my destination.

One man, who had just got off a plane, ran up to a woman, I'm presuming his wife or girlfriend. I expected them to latch onto one another and spin in circles, but as he got closer, he stopped.

They exchanged an uncertain glance and then decided to throw caution to the wind and embraced.

What a strange time we live in, I thought, and kept walking down the aisle toward my gate.

Before I knew it, I had reached my gate. The plane was already outside and apparently waiting on us.

I looked around and noticed there weren't many people waiting, maybe a dozen or so, and we only had about fifteen minutes left until we were supposed to board.

That's when a little boy with a red ball cap caught my eye. They weren't wearing a mask which alarmed me. By now, I would hope that everyone understood the efficacy of masks, but that was hardly the case.

He was playing on his mom's phone completely immersed in whatever it was he was doing. He was probably watching a YouTube video or playing a game or something.

I don't have any kids. I haven't given it much thought, to be clear, but maybe one day God will see fit to put the right person in my life, and we'll have some kids of our own. I do like kids, though. But the timing isn't right yet. Not to mention, with this career of mine, I couldn't imagine trying to introduce a child into that equation. I'm gone all the time, working.

I think it's the innocence of children that I appreciate the most. Life hasn't hardened them like it has you and I, and that I have a sincerity about them that's impressive. Makes you wish you capture whatever ingredient they have, bottle it up, and use it for yourself.

"Mom, when do I have to go back to school?" he asked.

"Not until next year," his mom said, patting him on the head.

I smiled at the little guy who shot me a glance. He didn't seem to mind that they wouldn't be back in school, physically, for some time. He still should have had on a mask though.

Eventually, we boarded the plane, and I was happy to see that I had a window seat. I've always preferred the window seats.

When the same little boy and his mom passed me in the aisle later on their way to their seats, we exchanged another nod. This time I was looking at his mom like c'mon lady where is his mask?

That's why I do what I do. Not to be cheesy or anything like that – but I do like helping people. I like seeing people happy and healthy and not having to worry about things like coronaviruses and other crappy illnesses.

I did dread this flight, though, and my stomach was already growling for food. Plus, in my experience, you'd be happy to grab a bag of peanuts or something in route and certainly not enough to hold you over.

We had two layovers. To make a longer story short, the rest of the trip went off without a hitch. I don't know where that little boy went – but I pray his mom got him a mask eventually. Kids are not immune to Covid-19.

. . .

When I stepped off the plane in Seattle, I realized that my phone had been in my pocket for some time. It was showing almost a dozen missed messages, which was bizarre to say the least.

Nonetheless, I was starving by that point, and I just wanted to get to my rental car, so that I could grab some food and then head over to the hotel to get some rest.

And then the phone rang once more. It was my recruiter on the other end. I couldn't imagine what he wanted.

"James, why haven't you answered your phone?" he shouted.

"I've been on a plane that you booked for me by the way. We just landed, and I need to go grab some food. I'm starving."

"Well, hold up a minute. There's been a change of plans."

"What's going on?"

"Are you sitting down?"

"Not hardly. But go ahead."

"Well, there's been a big mix-up, man. I'm sorry."

"What do you mean, 'mix-up?'"

"Your temp license!" he shouted. "It's been terminated."

My heart sank.

What on earth is he talking about? I wondered.

I was thoroughly confused. It was a new gig. The license was fine. I was all good to go. Hell, they are the ones who set this all up. I only paid for the flight and car, which was supposed to be reimbursed.

My blood pressure was raging at that point. Mind you, I'm not normally an angry person, but this was ridiculous.

"I just flew across the country, and I'm just now hearing about this?"

"Look, I'm sorry. But you're not going to be able to work there, okay? Plus, they're now saying they're overstaffed anyway."

"Overstaffed? Are you kidding me?" I shouted and then looked around instinctively because I knew I was losing my cool right there in the middle of the airport, which isn't a good thing.

Nonetheless, my futile attempts to contain myself quickly failed. I was raising my voice at the manager, which was completely beyond my norm. I don't know if it was my venting that helped or the fact that an airport security guard was now eyeballing me – but suddenly, a calm started to fall over me.

Now, I happen to be a rather large, towering black man in an airport, and there I was screaming at my phone like some lunatic. In today's uber-sensitive world, that's enough to get you in trouble, so maybe that's what it was. Or maybe I was already trying to figure out my next steps.

I rushed over to a bench to try to process the information and let my blood pressure go back down.

But before I knew it, I was bombarding the man on the other end of the phone with questions.

"Why didn't they just tell you this the other day? And who is reimbursing me for this flight? And where do I go from here?" I added, gesturing with my arm raised high into the air.

The hunger pains were more than I could handle by then, too, which contributed to my shitty attitude.

So, I started looking around the airport for the nearest chicken sandwich and cold, sweet tea.

Mind you, I am a vegetarian. But suddenly, I had a hankering for chicken if you can believe that. I know, it surprised the hell out of me, as well.

Come to think of it, they say people eat their feelings. I now believe that's true because I was ready to eat some serious quantities of grub, and by grub, I mean animal protein.

Anyway, after the fiftieth apology, he finally said he had a plan, and I was thankful to hear that because my nerves were holding on by a thin thread at that point.

He explained that he could get me to New York if that's what I still wanted, and my eyes must have bulged out of my head.

New York? I thought, smiling, as a new calm washed over me.

"Look, I was just informed that they are actually waiving their license requirements as long as you have one from another state, which you do," he explained.

"That's what I wanted," I said.

"That is what you wanted," he added. "Not to mention, they also happen to be paying people top dollar right now because they are in desperate need for help, especially people with your skillset."

I was happy all over again – but there was one lingering concern. But he beat me to the thought.

"Oh, by the way," he added. "We will be paying your travel expenses, so don't worry about that. You'll get your money back soon."

Hell yea! I thought. *That's what I wanna hear!*

Like I said before, I don't know if it was divine intervention or the fact I was so upset they knew they had to find some way to appease me. I choose to think the former versus the latter.

So, I jokingly told him to toss in a chicken sandwich and some iced tea, and we had a deal.

"Deal!" he interjected. "Just keep your receipts."

"Perfect. I'll see how quickly I can get myself to New York," I added and hung up the phone.

Do you remember that old cartoon called Carmen Sandiego? That's what I felt like. They had me flying all over the place. I had gone all the way across the country before finding out I needed to come back the opposite direction, and it wasn't on one of those first-class jumbo jets either. Not hardly.

After we got off the phone, I was finally able to fulfill my hunger pains. I made my way to a restaurant, scarfed it down so fast I'm not sure if I chewed, and then pulled up flight info for New York City on my phone.

Let me just iterate we have all seen the newsreels. But in all honestly, even though I wanted it, I had no idea what I was about to get into.

I have undoubtedly seen some things as an RT. I've planned, and I've studied, and I've prepared. But nothing can prepare you for what was going down in New York at that time. And it's a miracle I even made it there.

Chapter 4

A Ghost Town

To my astonishment, they had another flight going to New York City within the hour. While I waited, my appetite already satiated, I pulled my phone back up and started reading again.

For some context, earlier this year, New York had become the first epicenter in the United States for the novel coronavirus outbreak, which has killed well over 100,000 people in this country as of the time of the writing of this book and left many thousands more infected with the virus.

Hope has started to return to the Big Apple, and the whole of the Empire State, since the time I went there, but at the time try to picture what was going on.

They went from the worst infection rate in the entire nation to the best infection rate. I like to think thanks to people like me and other frontline works who dawned their PPE and went into a warzone for lack of a better word.

The very first confirmed case in that state was on March 1, and not too long afterward they went into a state of lockdown. In fact, it wasn't until June 8 they had a partial reopening of New York City.

On March 2, the governor of that state, Mario Cuomo, met with the mayor of New York City, Bill de Blasio. The two men promised to work together and perform contract tracing beginning with the area's first known case (or patient zero who was reportedly a lady who had recently traveled from Iran).

On March 5, Gov. Cuomo announced that statewide cases had doubled overnight from just 11 to 22. On March 6, cases doubled again to 45. And on March 8, New York reported 105 cases, doubling again.

By that point things were really ramping up, so the governors of New York, New Jersey and Connecticut agreed on March 16 to formulate the same rules for closures, saying they were forced to act because of a lack of coordination from the feds.

Soon afterward, on March 18, the governor signed an executive order that mandated all but essential business to reduce their work density by half and have more people work from home. New York cases hit 3,437 on that day. That's over 300 times the amount of cases in less than two weeks if you're keeping up.

On March 19, cases eclipsed 4,000. That's when the governor scaled the work density mandate to no more than 25% of a company's regular workforce. The state was also recording record overnight testing, which sent the statewide figure to 5,638. And the very next day, he ordered all nonessential businesses closed statewide.

Needless to say, when I flew into New York City, the order had already taken effect. That same order also barred all non-elective surgeries, and by the time it became active on the 22nd, statewide cases had surpassed 8,000.

New York City surpassed 12,000 cases on the 23rd, which represented about 35% of all Covid cases in the U.S. at that time, a pretty astounding figure.

I don't want to bog you down with too many more numbers, but suffice it to say, cases kept soaring from there. We've all seen the headlines.

On March 29, cases totaled 59,513. And there were 965 deaths related to Covid at that time in the city.

When I made it to John F. Kennedy airport, it looked like one of those Old West ghost towns you see at the theatre. While there was no tumbleweed, it was almost entirely devoid of human beings. I might have walked by ten employees at the most the whole time.

What few people I did see were all wearing masks, had very little to say, and mostly just kept their heads down. I got the impression they thought they could get Covid by looking at someone. I don't know.

I finally stopped and asked one of them where everyone was at.

"This is it," he shrugged. "There is a global pandemic going on, you know?"

"I know," I quipped and continued walking. I didn't see the need to go into any detail why I was there.

I followed the signs to the car pickup spot when fear started to set in. I found myself beginning to seriously second guess my choice to hop on a flight to New York. I mean, this was early-April, which was ground zero for the coronavirus pandemic in this country at that point.

What am I doing here? Do I really want to help? I wondered.

Then the thought of contracting the virus and dying hit me. To be honest, up until then, it's just not something I thought a lot about. But I wasn't in a hotspot like New York City either.

All these questions – and fears – were racing through my mind as I twirled my hair (it's an old nervous habit that's hard to break).

From what I read, nearly 5,000 members of the NYPD were out sick with about 900 having tested positive for the virus.

New York cases hit 75,795 by the end of March with 1,941 deaths.

In one damn month the entire state of New York went from a single case on March 1 to more than 83,000 statewide and more than 2,300 dead on April 1. What's worse, by April's end, the virus would claim another 16,000 lives across the state, many of those right there in the hospital I worked at.

I know. It's a lot to take in. Now, imagine you are there in the middle of it. And I had this impression that my goal of coming to New York was turning into a nightmare.

My heart was racing, and I had a lump in the back of my throat. That's the universal sign that you're about to cry by the way. Thoughts of my family back home slipped in. I didn't know if I was going to see them again.

The money was nice, but I was now questioning if it was worth it or not. I also questioned whether or not I was going to be helpful to the people there – or if it was a childlike fantasy I had somehow concocted to make myself feel better.

I'm not a psychologist, but it's been said that your mind will start playing tricks on your whenever you're in an uncomfortable or uncertain situation. To put this in no uncertain terms: I was getting mind fucked. Fear had set-up shop in my brain and was having a damn field day.

When I jumped in the back of the Uber, we barely exchanged a word at first. I was impressed with the truck he was driving, though.

It was a rather clean, obsidian black 2020 Ford Expedition. The funny thing is, it almost reminded me of a hearse – or else that was my mind playing more tricks on me. He also had this huge plastic shield separating the front seat from the back seat.

I noticed where it was starting to fall in places – and he didn't have a mask on either, but I didn't say anything.

He seemed incredibly nervous, too, like he didn't know if he should be out there either. But you have to make money somehow, right?

I thought about telling him about myself, my job, why I was here, and all those things, but then I hesitated. Why bother?

Keep it to yourself. Don't scare the non-medical professionals, I thought.

But then he ended up breaking the ice, which was nice, because one thing I've noticed from all of this is that I'm a people person and starve for human connections which I'm not getting during the virus.

"Wha, wha, what brings you to New York," he said, shuttering.

"My flight was canceled until tomorrow," I said, lying. "So, I'm staying overnight. I'll be gone soon."

"Yo! That sucks, bruh. You see how it is out here? It's not the place to be for anyone. I don't know why I'm still here," he asked, pointing out the window at the sheer nothingness around us.

"I was just thinking to myself how empty it is out there, too. This shit looks fucking scary. I'm not gonna lie," I admitted.

He let out a deep sigh and paused.

"It's not the same city anymore, man," he said. "The only things open are pizza spots and Bodegas, and you have to get your shit to go. Most people are out of work altogether. I guess you can call me one of the lucky ones, but I don't feel so lucky.

42

"Yea, I know what you mean," I replied.

"I shouldn't complain," he added, starting to feel more comfortable with my presence, I imagined. "I'm just glad I'm still working," he said as he flipped the blinker and prepared to turn onto 38th avenue.

"That's crazy, bro," I said, looking around in shock. "Nothing like I remember," I added, marveling out the window. It was a total ghost town.

I thought about the millions of people who lived in and around New York City. Millions of people commuted into and out of the city on any given normal day. The streets are packed with people from all over the world.

Time Square is like an event all unto itself.

Of course, that was before Covid happened. In one short month, they went from 1 case to over 80,000 throughout the state.

Needless to say, the whole city had changed. Millions of peoples' lives were on hold. Businesses were shuttered. Streets were empty. No busses were running. No cars were packed into the streets like sardines. No angry motorists were yelling at each other with the occasional middle finger. No bike messengers were zipping in and out of traffic. No food carts were peppering the sidewalks. No concession stands were selling over-priced magazines, knock-off Gucci, and loose cigarettes.

As a matter of fact, I didn't even see any homeless people, so they may have found somewhere to go. I'm still not sure.

No doubt, it was a sight to behold. This was not the city I had grown accustomed to seeing. It felt like a foreign land whose inhabitants had long ago deserted for better places.

On the bright side, what would have normally taken twenty-five minutes to get to the hotel only took us about five minutes to get there.

After our brief conversation, the driver pulled to an abrupt stop and shot me a glance in the rearview mirror.

"Hey, thanks for the ride. I really appreciate it, dude," I said and stepped away from the big, black hearse to grab my things.

He shot me a salute with a "no problem," and he was off again, slowly disappearing down the desolate street.

I looked up at the big sign on the front of the hotel. This was going to be my home for a little while, so whatever is going on in there, I tried to tell myself, I better get used to it quickly.

. . .

When I walked inside, the hotel attendant looked at me like I was the first person she'd encountered in a while. I probably was.

It made me wonder if maybe I had food on my face or something stuck in my teeth, but then I quickly remembered what was going on. It's just so hard to get used to how different things were.

"Welcome!" she said with the world's biggest smile on her face. "Are you checking in?" she added, putting me at calm.

"Yes," I replied and reached for my wallet.

She leaned into the counter, grinning.

"I just need an ID and a credit card for the incidentals."

"No problem."

I fumbled through my stuff and eventually found what I was looking for. To be honest, I am always losing things. I'm the world's biggest clutz. So, I'm glad I didn't leave anything important behind like licenses, money, etc.

That's when she scratched her head and started looking like something was troubling her.

"It says you're here for 13 weeks? Is that right?"

"Yup. I'm going to be working here at a hospital to help out," I blurted, not thinking.

That was a big mistake.

Her face dropped. The big smile that once dawned her face was now gone. She dropped my driver's license, slowly backed away, and acted like she couldn't pick it up anymore.

She took her huge gulp instinctively as if to try to swallow the invisible knot in the back of her throat.

What did I do? I wondered. I mean, I am a tall, somewhat menacing looking guy, I suppose. But I wouldn't hurt a fly, and moments ago she was just as happy as she could be.

"Hospital?" she said.

Oh, that's it, I thought.

She must think I have or will have the zombie apocalypse.

She finally managed to pick up my ID and place it on the counter before taking a huge step backwards again.

I don't even know if she realized how she was acting, but I certainly noticed. Truthfully, it was impossible not to. She was already six feet away, and now she was about eight feet away.

Without speaking, she backed away even further and then disappeared into a side room.

I was left standing there as if I had done something wrong, which was incredibly awkward to say the least.

Several minutes must have passed. The whole time I'm thinking how hungry I am again. It had been hours since that chicken sandwich, and I was growing very hungry once again.

When she finally returned, she had a stack of towels and some facecloths.

"All medical workers get extra towels because we are only turning over rooms once a week unless you call. It's the new protocol."

She disappeared again and came back with two key cards.

"Your room is on the 9th floor," she added and walked away without another word. It was all very cold and transactional.

Obviously, no bellhop was going to be tending to my bags or anything like that, which is perfectly fine by me. I was just ready to get to the room and find something to snack on before hitting the sack.

When I got in the elevator I was still in disbelief. I mean, you would have thought I was a walking, talking virus. I understand that people have to take precautions, but there's a right way and a wrong way to do that.

It's not that I took it personally. Not at all. People tend to fear what they don't understand. So, I vowed to be cordial, nonetheless, when I met her again, which I certainly would.

When I made it to my room, I scarfed down some crappy cereal bars I had stored away in my bags. I was thankful for them, because I didn't want to trouble the Uber driver with stopping so I could grab some takeout on the way to the room. I'm not that picky anyway.

That first night, I didn't bother to unpack either. I was too tired for all of that. It's weird how I had made it to New York City.

46

It was a very out of the way path to say the least having flown all the way to Seattle first only to find out I was no longer needed there.

I don't even remember closing my eyes that first night in the hotel. But at some point, I fell asleep with my clothes on as the hoopla from the day slowly faded away.

Chapter 5

A Distinct Smell

I had switched to working nights for a little while in the days leading up to my trip to New York, so when I found out I would be working days, I was partly relieved but partly worried, too.

It would take me several days to get settled back into the new normal and get my days and nights switched back around. If you've ever worked night shifts, you sleep during the day in rooms that you try to black the light out as much as possible. I know I can't sleep with the least little bit of light on, so when the sun shined through my blinds that first morning in the city, I woke up instantly. The alarm clock hadn't even rung yet.

I walked past a new attendant at the desk that morning and we exchanged some pleasantries. I'm glad to report that this dude didn't treat me quite as coldly as the lady from the night before.

"What brings you here?" Sam asked (I've changed his name for the purpose of this story).

I hesitated momentarily to tell him what I was doing here. After last night, I figured anyone I told my real reason for coming would treat me like an alien with a nasty virus.

But something about lying just doesn't feel right even when the ends otherwise justify the means.

"I'm a Respiratory Therapist, and I'm here to help out at one of the hospitals."

His eyes lit up, which caused me to delight in his presence. Finally, someone was treating me like I was used to.

He explained to me how bad things had gotten in the area recently.

I mean, I had read plenty about what New York was going through before I came, but until you come and before you speak with the people there, it's hard to get a good idea for how badly things were going at the time.

"You know what gets me?" he added.

"Nah. I don't. What's that?" I asked, grinning. I also asked myself whether he was flirting, a nasty habit. I needed to concentrate.

"I haven't seen my mom in weeks."

"Oh, I'm sorry to hear that," I said.

"I just worry that I might spread it to her," he admitted.

"That's probably smart," I added. "Especially if she has any pre-existing conditions. We're learning more about the virus all the time, but there are certain issues that seem to be a major factor."

"Do you mind sharing more with me about it?"

"You know," I said, leaning in. "I don't mind at all. Tell you what, I'm kind of running late. I really need to catch my ride over to the hospital, but I'd be glad to share my experiences with you soon."

"That'd be nice," he said. "Hope this whole thing goes away soon."

"Me too. And hey, don't forget to keep wearing your mask. And in the meantime, maybe call your mom," I added and headed for the door.

It would be a couple of days before I caught up with Sam again, and I finally made sure I had enough time to tell him about some of the things to look out for when it comes to the virus.

For some context, what we now call Covid-19 is a respiratory condition caused by a coronavirus, which is a family of viruses related to the cold. But it's nothing like the common cold – or the flu – and I hate when I hear people try to compare it to those things.

There are some pretty nasty symptoms for Covid, but some people who get infected don't actually notice any symptoms. But that doesn't mean they are infectious.

Most people will, in fact, have only mild symptoms and get better on their own without the help of medical care. But approximately 1 in 6 people who get the virus will have severe problems, such as trouble breathing.

The odds of having more serious symptoms get higher the older you are or when accompanied by another health issue like diabetes or heart disease.

We don't know everything we'd like to know about the virus, but there are generally some things to look out for if you think you may have Covid-19.

Some of the main symptoms include: fever, fatigue, dry cough, loss of appetite, body aches, shortness of breath, sore throat, headache, chills, shaking, loss of smell or taste, congestion, runny nose, nausea, vomiting, diarrhea, trouble breathing, pain or pressure in the chest, bluish lips, sudden confusion, and mucus or phlegm.

And symptoms tend to begin about 2 to 14 days after coming into contact with the virus from what I know thus far.

It's like I always tell people, if you have any of these more severe symptoms, never hesitate to get medical care as soon as possible.

During these times, that can even be tricky, but you can at least call your doctor's office or hospital before going in, so they can get prepared to treat you and protect medical staff and other patients.

. . .

My uber driver shot across the city in no time and had me in front of the hospital within a few short minutes.

When we pulled up, I will never forget what I saw: we passed two freezer trucks that were parked outside, waiting to carry the dead bodies away, when we arrived.

I still recall seeing the same type of trucks in Italy weeks ago on the television. I remember thinking how awful that must be to have to resort to those tactics, and I prayed that we would never get to that point in this country. Yet here we were.

I exchanged a quick glance with the driver. I think we were both thinking the same thing. Something like, "This is really messed up." But we didn't say anything. There's nothing really to say when you see something like that.

It's horrific.

As I walked up to the hospital I tried to forget about the trucks, but it was impossible. I once again questioned what I was doing there.

You see this stuff on TV, but nothing can prepare you for what was happening there.

When I got inside, a familiar smell hit my nostrils just before I put my scarf back on. I took it off for one second to readjust it.

Death.

It has a distinct smell to it. Anyone who has ever been around a dead body can attest to that.

I approached the security desk to ask for help.

"All travelers, please get in the temporary badge line to my left," he yelled over the muffled crowd voices.

There was so much confusion. It didn't seem like anything was organized at all, just pure pandemonium.

"I'm looking for the Respiratory Department," I said, so he could hear me over the crowd of people.

"Are they expecting you?" he questioned me.

Why wouldn't they be? Do people just visit random departments? I wondered.

The security guard finally motioned me in line when he was interrupted by what looked like a visitor. He seemed burnt out and annoyed by everyone.

In the line, there were people covered from head to toe. They had on so much personal protective equipment that all you could see was their eyeballs.

Where's my suit? I wondered, twisting my dreadlock again. That's one nervous tick that's hard to shake.

All I had was a peace sign scarf that was wrapped so tightly around my face that I could barely breathe, but I knew that wasn't going to handle what I needed.

Everyone else looked like they had just stepped out of the movie, "Twelve Monkeys."

The lobby was jam-packed with people, and I got the impression that a lot of us were travelers, so I wasn't alone in this strange, new environment.

"Are you a traveler?" I asked an older woman behind me.

"Yea, I'm from Alabama," she said, adjusting her mask. "I drove up with two other nurses last night."

Her surgical gown almost swallowed her shoes. She was so tiny and had so much PPE on.

"Wow!" I said in disbelief. I shuffled out of the line to let someone go by and returned to my spot.

"That is a long ass drive," I acknowledged.

She looked over her goggles.

"It really was, but I wanted a car. I didn't know how the public transportation system would be."

"I flew in yesterday but got an Uber this morning. I'm getting a rental tomorrow because I'm not going to pay for rides every day."

She nodded in agreement.

"I get it completely. I have a whole family back down my way. But I wanted to help out any way that I could and make some extra money to support my kids. I'm scared, but I feel like God has my back."

That poor mask kept falling down her tiny face every time she spoke, and she struggled to continuously adjust it.

"I think you need a new mask, hun," I teased.

We exchanged some more small talk, and then the line began to move again.

"Well, you be safe. You need to get home to your family," I said as we moved forward.

"Same to you, my friend. Maybe I will see you around," she said, holding her mask onto her face.

"You will definitely be seeing me around. "I'm respiratory."

She placed her hand over her heart.

"God bless you! Good for you, young man. That is a tough job, and it's needed now more than ever. I couldn't do it, but I am glad some people can," she added.

"Thank you!" I said, looking down at my feet. "I just want to help. Same as you."

From other quick conversations in line, I gathered no one knew what to expect. People were scared and nervous. Some were happy and eager to help while others wanted a paycheck.

Some people had many years of experience, while others had barely any experience whatsoever.

Our little line was a hodgepodge of different professions, experiences, skillsets, and backgrounds.

Please don't let the newbies in the Intensive Care Unit, I thought. Sometimes, I can't help myself, but it's true. I would not want them to take care of my parents. Not during a pandemic.

The feeling in the lobby was very tense. You could feel the nervousness radiating off of the people. That alone was giving me anxiety, too. I am what's often called an empath, so I very strongly feel what other people feel.

I think that is why I always try to make people happy. If I made them happy, I won't have to deal with their heavy negative emotions. I'm getting better at letting people just be though. Sometimes people need to deal with their own feelings.

The atmosphere could only be described as complete chaos. People were asking for directions. People were looking for different units and departments. Managers were walking around, going over agency names. Some employees were being ushered toward the elevators in a single file line. It looked like Prefects leading students to their dormitories in the Harry Potter saga.

While in the badge line, I caught myself tearing up because there were family members begging security officers to let them into the lobby to see their loved ones.

"Just let me see him for a second," someone shouted.

"I just want to make sure they are ok," one person pled.

"Don't kill him," an older Spanish-speaking lady said.

That's when I realized that all visitation was banned. It's not that I don't understand because I do. It's for their own safety. We have to minimize the exposure to the public, which was already rampant.

I couldn't imagine not being able to see my sick loved ones when they were dying. That had to be terrifying.

It took everything in my power to not scream with the crowd, "Hey, just let them in for a few minutes!" But as a medical professional, I understand why the rules are in place the way they are.

I had the thought that maybe they could gown up and go seem them at their own risk. I ended up stepping out of the badge line and walking over to the Spanish woman who was hysterical at this point.

I introduced myself in Spanish and asked her who she wanted to see and when was the last time she saw them. She explained to me it was her husband. She had called over one hundred times, and no one would update her. They just kept telling her that they would call her back and never did. Security was telling her the same thing now. She would just have to keep calling.

I was starting to get a handle on the magnitude of the problem. But now that there were more reinforcements, it was unacceptable to me what was happening with this person.

I asked the security guard where the administration office was. He had pointed to a lady and told me that she was a boss. After a five-minute conversation we were able to find a resolution.

As it turns out, the woman's husband was not on a vent, and they were going to set up a device so he could FaceTime with her.

So, I hadn't even started my job, and I was already helping, which made me feel a little bit better.

While I was there, I was always stumbling into something. Anytime I saw someone in need, my spirit got super uneasy until I was able to help.

It took a while longer, but eventually, I got my badge. You couldn't get in and out of the building without one.

After that, I received my N95 mask. This is an extremely specific type of mask to protect us from the virus. But I was told not to throw it away and to save it for at least three or four days.

Of course, my jaw dropped almost instantly. My eyes bugged wide open in disbelief. These masks are designed for one-time use only. Usually, you're supposed to change your mask every time you enter a patient's room. Even if it's the same patient, you're supposed to change it every time you go inside.

At first, I figured hey, they're probably joking. It is the fact we use PPE and are so sterile in how we do things nowadays that we have made such tremendous strides in health care.

So, I informed him that he must have lost his mind if he thought I was going to reuse this same mask for three or four days.

I asked him if he had any patient contact at all. He replied he didn't. I told him he could reuse his mask all he wanted, but I was coming back the next day and every day afterward for a new one. I don't know who he thought I was, but homie don't play that. Period!

"Good for you," an older guayanese woman who was behind me said.

As I walked out, I went down the line and told everyone to not listen to him and to get a new mask every day. I was not going to catch this virus because someone wanted to play "mask police." Our safety was important too.

I eventually made my way up the elevator to the Respiratory Department. Before getting there, the elevator stopped at almost every floor with several people getting on and off.

When the doors opened, I peered into the hallway. All you could see was a flood of blue gowns rushing back and forth. I heard unanswered call bells and Code Blues over the loudspeakers.

I must have heard Code Blue called seven or ten times on my way up the elevator alone. I assumed it was for the same patient, and the chaos was preventing people from hearing what was happening.

I was wrong.

I later found out that were several different people in cardiac arrest at that exact same time, but we will get into more of that later.

I walked into the Respiratory Department. There was a bathroom just outside. I dashed in and took three deep breaths. I looked in the mirror and tried to convince myself I had this.

Remember why you're here, I thought.

A sudden calm rushed over my entire body. The panic melted away. And I hoped beyond hope that everything was going to be ok. I also the feeling I was somehow safe and being protected if that makes any sense.

I believe in guardian angels, and my guardian angel was about to put in some overtime.

After the little pep talk, I snapped into work mode and burst into the Respiratory Department with my head held high.

Let the madness begin, I thought.

Chapter 6

Dressed for War

I have never been a shy person. So, when I walked into the department, I greeted everyone. I was met by a super, pleasant young lady named Ydna. She seemed really leveled headed and calm.

I instantly gravitated to her. She introduced me to the Director, who was very pleasant, as well. You could tell she had a tough side. I can read people well, and something told me she was not the one to be messed with. It was written all over her face. She could smile and glare all at the same time, which is an impressive feat.

I call it "gliling."

Thankfully, she assigned the young woman I just met to be my preceptor. I guess you could say that's the person who takes you under their wing.

I was then told to wait until the report was finished, and I would get squared away with all of my PPE.

As I sat, I took in the room. It was filled with tons of RTs. It was mixed with day and night shift people. The night shift was the ones taking off their personal protective equipment and getting ready to leave.

They looked exhausted.

I saw them wiping all their stuff down as they gave reports and handed off their patients to the day-shifters.

They wiped down their sneakers, cellphones, pens, badges, keys. Everything. They clearly meant business and were not taking any chances. That gave me a sense of calm.

After the report was finished and the night shift went home, I finally received my PPE. I had an operating room gown, covers for my shoes, a bouffant for my hair, the N95 for my face, and a big, clear shield for my eyes.

It felt like I was putting my wardress on. In no time, I was hot and uncomfortable. I was sweating my balls off and could barely breathe with the mask on my face.

Remember, those masks were originally designed for one-time use. Typically, you wear it while you're in the patient's room and take it off when you leave.

This time was different. We had to wear these things everywhere we went all day long.

Soon afterward, I received the fastest tour in the history of tours. The entire tour of the hospital included only the most important places like the CT-scan and X-ray rooms. Each floor looked the same to me anyway. And I met several people throughout the viewing of the hospital, but it only took about ten minutes from start to finish.

I knew I wasn't going to remember anyone because they were also wearing PPE. I had no idea what anyone looked like. On top of that, their voices were muffled. Even though I didn't remember half of the stuff I was shown, I was a big boy and knew how to use my words if I needed directions later anyway.

After the tour, I was eager to get to work. Ydna said I was the fourth or fifth person she had trained, and she seemed annoyed by that.

She made small comments about the people she trained. Some were lazy. Some were stupid. I didn't hear any good comments, to be frank.

I told her I knew my shit, and she didn't have to worry. I proudly informed her that I started out at a Level 1 Trauma Center with some of the best healthcare professionals in the world. Was I the greatest? No! But I could certainly hold my own.

With that statement, she shot me a "we will see" expression. I guess I don't blame her.

She told me that she had the main ICU for an assignment by herself on top of having to precept me. I told her to just show me where the supply room was and that I could do the rest.

A hospital is a hospital, no matter where you go. I knew how to do my job. All I needed to know was where the respiratory equipment was.

I also asked her how many patients on vents she had because we could split them. A ventilator is used for life support. In short, it does the breathing for those who can't do it for themselves. We had twenty-four people on vents on our floor my first day.

Mind you, a normal vent to RT ratio is about six to eight vents per one RT. On a normal day, that is completely manageable. Twenty-four was not manageable for even two people. But I took twelve vents on one side, and she took twelve on the other.

Game on.

. . .

I quickly began my rounds. I checked on my patients. When I got to my first room, I noticed there were four patients inside. And each patient was on a vent. I could also see the vent alarms were going off on all of my patients.

I couldn't hear them because the doors were closed so the virus couldn't spread. Most vents display highlighted messages in different colors for when they alarm. As I peeked in, I saw reds and yellows. To put that in perspective, yellow means you need to get in there quickly, and red means you should already be in there.

As I entered, I saw right away that one of my patients had gotten accidentally disconnected from the vent. This happens for sometimes. The most common reason is that the patient pulls themselves off it.

When patients are on certain medications, they sometimes get really confused and have no control over their actions. Mix that with fear and the fact everyone around them looks like they were pulled from the movie, "Outbreak," and you get the drift.

You can also cough so hard if you have tons of secretions that if the connection is not tight for any reason, some of the tubing will pop loose. It happens, but there is always supposed to be someone in the room, outside the door, or close by to watch the monitor and listen for the alarms.

The front desk even has a monitor where you can see the patients' vitals. Some of the rooms also have cameras where you can see the patient from the front desk. This feature comes in handy when you have confused patients who sometimes end up climbing out of their beds.

I connected my patient back to their vent, and I checked and made sure everything was working properly. I notated all the alarms on their machine and turned the volumes all the way up to the max so I could hear the alarms better.

After the first patient, I moved on to the others. I checked them and their machines. I also turned their alarms up, as well.

All the patients were on a lot of oxygen. If you're maxed out on oxygen, it means you are on 100%. Oxygen goes from 21% to 100%. 21% is normal. That is what normal everyday people breathe. People who get sick or have a lung disease sometimes require more oxygen. In that instance, they all are extremely sick.

It took me about 3 hours to check all of my patients and make sure they were safe in the first round. I checked and tripled checked to make sure their machines were working properly. I made sure their breathing tubes were in the right places. I made sure they were all secure so they would be safe. I looked over their x-rays and lab work to make sure the vents were doing their jobs.

After I was done, I went to look for the nurse or nurses who were taking care of the patients. We needed to have a conversation.

Now, I love my nurses, and I get that sometimes they get busy and pulled away from their rooms, but at least have someone look out for your patients if you aren't going to be around. I understood we were in a crisis, but that's not the patients' fault, and that's why folks like me had been called in. We are there to help.

Some jobs have the luxury to allow for a certain level of mistakes, but healthcare is not one of those. Not when you're dealing with people's lives.

I asked several nurses in the hall if they had those patients. Every one of them said no. I eventually gave up and asked the secretary at the front desk.

By the way, the secretaries know everything! They know what nurses are assigned to what patients. They know what doctor is covering the floor. They know what CNAs are working the floor.

They know almost every phone number you would need to know in a hospital. They also know all the floor gossip that's going around, but that's a subject for another story.

The secretary informed me that the nurse was right outside her patient's room, the room I just left. I went over to the nurse and asked her if she was deaf. Now everyone who knows me, knows I love to joke around and have a good time.

I love to cheer people up when they are down. I hate seeing people upset. It's just something in me. I have always been like that.

But when it comes to my patients, I do not mess around. I'm not your friend at this point. I'm your co-worker. These are people's lives. You only get one chance to do this right. There are no "oops" moments allowed.

So, when it comes to patient safety, my delivery can be a little intense. She told me she was so caught up in her documentation that she didn't hear me.

Jen was a traveler, as well, and she was still trying to figure out how to put her patients' information in the computer system.

She looked so nervous and overwhelmed. She didn't know if she was coming or going. She said she had been so busy and was not used to this pace. I asked her how she would feel if that was her father on the vent, and he became disconnected. She didn't answer, but her face said it all.

She got the message. It's a very serious issue.

I couldn't stay mad for long, though. She was obviously exhausted. That could have very well been me in that same position.

It's so easy to judge people.

I actually think that most of us could do a better job of putting ourselves in other people's shoes. When we do that, our perspective inevitably changes.

I explained to her that it's important to at least face the room when you're busy with other tasks.

She ended up asking me some other questions about the vents, and I was more than happy to help her. And I noticed as she got better and better the whole time I was there.

However, my first day only got worse from there.

Chapter 7

Unfamiliar Faces

As the day progressed, I waited for a camera crew to jump out of a janitor's closet. I hoped that I was on a prank show, and at any moment someone was going to say, "Gotcha." Unfortunately, no one ever jumped out of the closet, and the situation only worsened.

I went to over 30 Code Blues and 30 rapid responses on my first shift. A Code Blue is called whenever someone is in cardiac arrest. A rapid response (or RRT) is called when a patient is in danger of cardiac arrest. Either way, both situations are very intense and require immediate attention.

During a Code Blue, everything happens very quickly. Everyone has a specific job to do, but the main goal is to save the patient. There is also normally someone recording everything that is going on, too.

At the same time, someone is overseeing medications. Other people are performing CPR. Respiratory is usually at the head of the bed, putting in a breathing tube, while the doctor is talking, keeping order, and giving clear instructions to everyone.

In an RRT, the patient is not in cardiac arrest but is still extremely sick and unstable. There will be a team trying to figure out what's going on, so they can stabilize the patient and avoid the "Code Blue" situation altogether. During these alarms, mostly, the same people are involved.

The doctor, the nurse, and the Respiratory Therapist attend the rapid response. There will also be X-ray, nursing assistants, and nursing supervisors as well, who do their parts.

So, everyone has a role, and everyone is essential in these situations, including phlebotomy. We need labs in these scenarios, so the phlebotomist (i.e., the vampires) are always there to help.

The whole day we just went to various Code Blues and RRT's. My feet still hurt thinking about it. Up and down the stairs. Back and forth down the halls. Up and down the stairs again.

Yes, they had an elevator, but those took way too long. Each time we got to the room during a Code Blue, it was the same story playing out over and over. It was a madhouse. Everyone is sweating under all their PPE. Their backs and arms are sore from doing CPR on all these patients.

Every time we got to a room for an RRT, the patient's oxygen saturation was low. Despite giving them 100%, they still had low oxygen. So, they would end up going on a vent, too.

Keep in mind, under normal circumstances, respiratory would try other things for patients with low oxygen before going to the vent, but most of those things spread throughout the air. They tried to use those devices in Italy, and a lot of their workers got infected and died as a result.

There was a rapid response I went to for a young black man. He was probably about 26. He had Covid, and we couldn't keep his oxygen up with the NRB mask. The doctor told him he needed to go on a ventilator.

He looked at me and asked me if he was going to die. I told him he was strong and going to be ok.

That's when he grabbed my hand and started to cry. He had no family with him, only us, a long line of doctors, RTs, CNAs, techs, phlebotomists, and other staff. All unfamiliar faces.

We tried to comfort him, but we are nothing but strangers when it comes right down to it. We can't replace the comfort and love of a close family member. It's truly heart wrenching.

He ended up calling his mother, who said a prayer for him on the speaker phone. I stayed with him while he spoke to her.

The truth was, I didn't know if he was going to be all right. Then, there was that lump again in my throat. I swear I'm a big cry baby sometimes.

The man was close to my age. It could have very well been me. I can only imagine the fear and anxiety he must have been feeling.

I wanted to cry with him. It took everything in me to hold back my tears. I have brothers and it could have very well been one of them in the same situation.

I ended up making some corny jokes before finally getting a laugh out of him to lessen the mood. It was all I could do to cheer him and give him some glimmer of hope.

I don't even know half the stuff I say. It's almost like something takes over and speaks for me. I always manage to find the right words at the right time, or I certainly try.

Shortly after the call, he hung up, and he was intubated by an anesthesiologist. Then I placed him on a ventilator. The good news is, I was able to get his oxygen up. And all went well. He was stable, and I was on to the next crisis.

Several Code Blues and rapid responses were called throughout the day. Some people survived, but a lot of people did not. Some of them I went to and some of them I did not. You cannot be everywhere at one time. The other RT's I worked with did an exceptional job with keeping up with all the codes. It was so amazing to see their teamwork and dedication. Most of them were overworked and tired but always pushed on. Shout out to them. But I digress.

I just hope this unfamiliar face was a comfort to the ones I did respond to and help. Anyway, that's some of the events that happened just on that first day.

I was so happy when the night shift crew came in, which was a sure-fire sign that it was our time to go home (or back to the room in my case).

I don't recall the ride home, but I will never forget the dream that I had that night. It would haunt me for some time.

Chapter 8

An Ominous Dream

After my first shift of working I was exhausted to say the least. Still yet, I must have tossed and turned for at least an hour before my body and mind eventually gave way to sleep. What happened next still disturbs me if I stop and really think about it.

At one point, I woke up to a loud noise and sat up quickly. At first, I felt like it must just be the trees whipping in the breeze, but then a strange sensation washed over my entire body.

In this dream-like state, I was in a cold place that was blacker than a moonless, overcast night. I was feeling my way forward as if I'd been stricken blind.

Where was I? I wondered.

I was completely lost and couldn't see where I was or where I was going.

Slowly, my eyes adjusted, and I realized I was back in my childhood bedroom at home, but it was much darker than normal. There was no window. I could hear distant conversations, almost whispers that were beyond my reach and completely lost amidst the darkness.

I hopped from my bed and worked my way slowly through the darkness and out into the hall.

In my constant anxiety, I was hoping for treasure, peace, tranquility. I was tired of the torment and just wanted a sweet peace, the kind that only comes from being completely comfortable with one's self and surroundings.

However, an uneasiness started to settle back in, and I could now see my own breaths in the cold air.

I knew I had to get out, so I continued to fumble through the nearly impenetrable darkness, feeling with my hands that were extended out in front of my face, moving this way and that. As I slowly moved forward, a subtle red glow pierced the darkness at the end of the hall.

Arms outstretched; I felt my way toward the light. The whole living room was now aglow with this red light as if it were guiding me. I could hear a piano playing in the distance, and I crept my way closer. There sat some stranger with his back to me attempting to play.

The hairs on my little arms stood at attention, and I finally bolted from the living room as this stranger, who kept his back to me, continued to pound away at the piano with not one ounce of discernible talent.

That's when I heard the laughter coming from what sounded like a crowed as I struggled to get away. I turned down the hall, but as I stepped forward it got longer and longer. There was no end in sight to the long corridor.

Frightened, I started to run as the piano kept playing the devilish tune and the laughter got stronger and stronger in the background.

The more I ran, the farther I got from my bedroom door, and I kept running and crying, trying to get away from the torment that their laughter represented.

I finally stopped in my tracks, ready to completely give myself up to whatever they wanted.

I fell to the floor when a familiar voice rang out.

It was my grandfather speaking to me.

74

"James, he said, come here young man. "What are you doing down there on the floor?"

My heart lit up as I looked up but couldn't find him.

"Grandpa?" I asked, looking around confused. I didn't see him. But my bedroom door was now within reach, so I jumped up and bolted inside.

I slowly caught my breath when I noticed a faint glow in the distance coming from outside the window.

There was a faint, red glow that was far away in the background, gently lighting the woods with an evil-red light. It got brighter and brighter until silhouettes of people in robes began to appear. They were marching around in perfect unison, and the laughter from earlier had returned.

The voices sounded familiar, but I couldn't make out who it was. All I could make out were their evil laughs as if taunting me.

Three of the glowing silhouettes finally stepped forward shoulder-to-shoulder and approached the window. No faces could be seen.

I stood petrified as these faceless beings approached. My throat started to tighten, and I gasped for air. Instinctively, I clenched at my throat as the air completely escaped me.

My heart was pounding.

It seemed like minutes before they moved, and then I started seeing them gather around the first three. Quickly, the middle one stepped forward and then thrust itself at the window.

I stumbled and fell backward but somehow managed to catch my fall. When I looked up, it's face was pressed hard against the glass.

Its eyes were glowing red, and its demonic face was twisted and distorted.

It opened its mouth so wide that all I could see was inside its mouth as the rest of its head disappeared. There were rows and rows of tiny, razor-sharp teeth, and it leaned back in toward the glass as my heart sank.

I had to escape.

I stumbled to my feet and then shot toward my door, but it was locked this time. I WAS SCARED BUT DEFINITELY WOULD HAVE FOUGHT WHATEVER THAT WAS.

I looked at my bed, which seemed much larger than normal and then ran and plunged into the sheets, but instead of landing in the warmth of my comforter, I was immersed in an icy pond.

My breaths had completely escaped me, and I stared up at the chunks of ice that were floating near the surface, as well as the faint, familiar red glow from the demon's torches in the background.

Oh my God, I'm drowning, I thought.

I can't breathe, I tried to scream, but my words failed me.

I wasn't going to give up, so I started beating at the ice with my hands, but the giant sheets would not break.

The silhouettes from outside had returned and were now moving around above me on the ice.

This is it. I'm going to die. No one can save me. Not even grandpa, I thought.

The life was pouring out of me as the water moved around my body.

I was slowly sinking further down until my feet finally hit the bottom of the pond.

There was one last glimmer of hope. I finally decided I was going to confront those evil things and take them down with me, so I started flailing my arms, trying to fight my way back to the surface.

When I finally reached the surface again, I reached for the ice and grabbed ahold, but it quickly broke free in my hand, and I started to sink again.

I felt the last bit of air in my lungs. If I was in a dream, I wanted someone to wake me from this horrible hell.

I stared up at the ice again with the distant haze of the red torches glowing in the distance. The water was so cold that my shaking finally ceased, and I felt completely frozen in terror.

One. Last. Scream, I thought and plunged back toward the surface in one last effort to emerge.

I roared and screamed as my head emerged from the icy pond.

I was safe and sound in my bed at the hotel. I looked around. The clock read 5 a.m.

Oh my God, I thought. *I am losing my mind.*

I tried to go back to sleep, but it was useless. In another hour or so the alarm was going to ring anyway, and I would be off to work.

I sat up in bed and thought about my dream. That horrible piano getting pounded in the background. Shadowy silhouettes attacking me. Glowing torches haunting my every thought.

But amidst all of that pain and torment I heard a familiar voice, my Grandpa. For that, I am thankful.

I went to the bathroom and turned the water as hot as I could stand it and got in.

As the water rinsed over my body images of the fiery torches continued to haunt me.

Chapter 9

Round Two

After that first day followed by an ominous dream that night, I can't say I rushed off to work eagerly. But something was pulling me that direction.

When I got to the hospital, I quickly dawned my PPE. If you're wondering, I didn't have any troubles getting a mask that morning or from there on out. I guess the guy who had been watching guard over them realized I wasn't going to start shifts without fresh gear.

I finally made my way back up to the Respiratory Department. I'd like to say that day two was better than one, but it was much of the same. I knew my way around better, but all the pain and struggle you see isn't something you just get used to really quickly.

The nightshift gave us their report and then parted way, and I eagerly rushed off to check on my patients. When I got to my first room, I noticed there were three patients inside. And one of them was on a vent. The vent alarms weren't all going off this time, so that was good.

I started to slowly make my rounds when we caught our first rapid response for the day. It was another black man. If I recall correctly, he was in his sixties.

He was new to my floor and had Covid, and we were having trouble keeping his oxygen up with the NRB mask, so the doctor wanted him placed on a vent.

He looked at me and asked me if he was going to die, and I didn't know what to tell him. I wanted to say, "Sure. You're going to be fine." But that feels so wrong, too, because in his case it wasn't looking good. So, I took the first chance I had to pat him on the arm and just let him know someone was there with him. He wasn't in this alone.

But what I didn't say, to him, was that he was in a battle with Covid and the virus was currently winning. Let me tell you what happens if you haven't seen this.

In most cases, the virus stays in the upper tract, which includes everything above the windpipe. In those cases, symptoms can include stuff as minor as a fever, cough or a sore throat, as we noted earlier.

The thing is, if the virus isn't considered severe, it hasn't entered the lungs. When it migrates to the lower tract, that's when the more severe symptoms like shortness of breath can occur and low oxygen levels.

In this man's case, the ventilator had to be used. Once the virus reached his lungs, it caused compounding issues including inflammation. He was already in heart failure so that didn't help either because fluid was backing up in his lungs. So, in other words, he was otherwise having difficulty breathing.

Unfortunately, in this case, the fluid filled the air sacs of his lungs, which was causing his blood oxygen level to also fall. On top of that he had pneumonia, a term most of you will be acquainted with.

Those air sacs are responsible for the much-needed gas exchange (that's the process of breathing in oxygen and breathing out carbon dioxide).

Obviously, we don't want this process to be interrupted, which is exactly what's happening with Covid in the more severe cases.

The cell disruption the virus causes in the lungs is the biggest reason why this illness causes such a severe respiratory pathology. That just means the behavior and characteristics of the disease.

Gas exchange is a critical and vital function to sustain human life. But that's the same function that the virus is disrupting.

So, the virus had entered his air sacs, where you can determine it interacts with a specific type of cell that lines the sacs. These are called the alveolar cells; specifically, they are called type II cells, to be precise.

That's actually how it got its name. The spike-like appearance of the coronavirus is how the illness interacts with a molecule on the type II alveolar cells. Think spike as in crown as in corona, which is the Latin word for crown or garland. If you didn't know, it's pretty neat how those names derive. But what's not neat is what this virus does to the human body.

It invades those cells, and once it gets inside them it starts to replicate and multiply and divide. It then creates copies of itself, and because it infects the one cell, that one cell essentially gets destroyed and bursts open.

When the cell bursts, it releases hundreds of new virus particles that will infect more and more cells, so the process just keeps going and going. It's highly effective as a killing machine.

Once the virus starts to destroy human cells that line the air sacs, how the immune system responds contributes to the difference between a person either recovering or dying.

That's why I like to know a patient's history as well as possible, too. I think about things like pre-existing conditions. Are they immuno-compromised? Age and certain pre-existing conditions can make a big difference between life and death.

In this man's case, we ascertained he had pre-existing conditions, and, at the same time, he was over sixty. And the virus was recking havoc on his system.

He was running a fever, which is good, because a person's immune system will respond to the virus by causing fever and inflammation

For some reason, in the U.S., the virus is killing Black Americans at a much higher rate than other races with Latinos in tow. It's like I said from the onset, Covid-19 is colorblind in that it's killing all manner of people; but like this man, it seems to favor darker skins tones for whatever reason.

You might say that systemic racism or lack of access to health care have made African Americans and Latinos more vulnerable to the virus, but those are subjects, perhaps, for another book.

When he grabbed my hand and started to cry I almost lost my control.

I may be a medical professional, but I'm also human, too, and that's something that tugs at you in ways you can't quite describe.

I wanted so badly to tell him everything would be okay.

When I looked into his eyes, I really saw flashes of my own grandpa, too, and that troubled me. But this man didn't have any family around to comfort him. We must tightly control visitors for obvious reasons. So, instead of family, he had nothing, but a long line of strangers faces such as myself, doctors, other RTs, RNs, CNAs, and others.

It's just a sea of unfamiliarity.

I can now report that he was still alive when I left my shift that evening – but I would never see him again. He didn't make it much longer, I'm sorry to say. But we tried our best.

I finally left the room to tend to my other patients.

When I entered the next room, there were four patients inside. I immediately saw that one of them had gotten accidentally disconnected from her vent. As noted, before, this happens for many reasons, but the most common reason is that the patient accidentally pulls it out themselves.

Sure enough, that's what happened. My next patient was a forty-something year old lady with a tan complexion. She was wide awake and fidgety on the vent.

She nodded at me as I fixed her tubes and reset the machine, and pretty soon, she was okay again. I started to move on to the next patient when she stopped me.

"Mmmmmbbb?"

"Ma'am? I'm sorry?"

I had no idea what she was talking about. She tried to mouth something. Patients who are awake enough try and speak, but it's impossible with the breathing tube going down their airway. I explained to her that she was ok and that she should get some rest.

I've seen a lot of sad situations before, but I couldn't imagine being on the other side of things (being in the hospital bed praying I see my loved ones one last time instead of helping them from our side).

Now add in an unhealthy amount of fear at having this strange virus, and it's a very alarming situation.

After conducting my rounds, I stopped at the front desk and chatted with the secretary briefly. But I made sure to never turn my back on my patients. Plus there's a monitor where you can see the patients' vitals right there at the desk.

While I chatted with the secretary, I started looking at one of the cameras which was of the inside of one of my rooms. That's when I noticed someone trying to climb right out of their bed, and I along with the nurse, bolted for their door.

As I burst through the door, my first instinct was to yell, "Wait!"

The old man stopped dead in his tracks and rolled over and looked up at me.

"What on earth are you yapping about?" he said.

He then verbally accosted me and the nurse like an old sailor in the Navy, but I didn't really mind. I was just happy he didn't fall onto the floor and hurt himself.

I quickly re-connected him to his oxygen, which he pulled off, and I checked and made sure that his oxygen saturation was ok.

I recalled his name from the chart.

"What are you trying to do in here Henry?"

"Oh, I was about to get me some exercise," he informed me.

"Is that right?"

"Yeah, that's right. Exercise is good for ya young man."

"Oh, I know, Henry. It sure is. And pretty soon, you'll be out this hospital and on your way home, so you can exercise all you want."

"That sounds really nice," he admitted, starting to calm down.

"I'm sure it does, Henry. I wish I could say it would be today or tomorrow, but it's hard to say."

Henry was one of my patients who was on a lot of oxygen.

He was actually maxed out at 100%, so we needed to get that down to around the twenties or so before he could even think about going home, much less exercise.

I tried explaining everything to him, but he seemed completely disinterested from what I was saying.

I started to leave when he caught my attention.

"What's your name by the way, kid?"

I spun around.

"James," I said, smiling.

"Well, you remind me of my grandson, James."

My heart sank. The poor guy was laying here with no family, not unlike all the others.

It was just a sea of humanity. And in this place you were either a patient or staff with very few exceptions.

"You miss your family?" I asked him before realizing that might have been a stupid question.

Who says that? I wondered. Of course, he misses his family.

"Yes, I do, James. Hey, you do me a favor, would you?"

"Anything, Henry. What can I do for you," I added, expecting him to ask for lunch or his nurse to bring him medication or something else.

He looked up to me in those dark, timeless eyes, windows to his soul, and uttered, "If you got somebody you love, make sure to tell 'em about it, okay?"

My heart dropped.

It was a simple yet profound statement. Henry had single handedly hit the nail on the head and brought to light the humanity that we all shared. This was the common link that connected all of us – doctors, staff, patients.

We're all human beings, and we all care deeply about loved ones, and we cannot take that for granted. I know these people certainly weren't while many of them were laying there dying without the very people around them they had spent a lifetime with.

It's incredibly sad.

I caught myself tearing up, when I wiped my eyes with the back of my hand and headed for the door. I tried to say thank you, but my voice cracked, and I walked out into the hall.

The thing is, I love to cheer people up when they are down. I hate seeing people upset. It's just something in me. I have always been like that. But this time the shoe was on the other foot. It was a patient who was encouraging me – and reminding me of what was important. Family.

. . .

It took me about 3 hours to check all my patients and make sure they were all safe and sound in my second round. I would check and then check again and make sure everything was working properly. Hey, it was just my second day, but I already felt like I had this under control.

As my day progressed, I attended so many Code Blues and rapid responses that it was hard to keep up.

During one Code Blue, everything happened so quickly that it's all still kind of a blur. As noted, before, everyone has a specific job to do, and the main goal of the whole team is to save the patient.

I rushed inside the room and took my position while someone else was overseeing medications. Someone else was already performing CPR on the patient, a young white man.

As the Respiratory Therapist, I was at the head, putting in the breathing tube, while the doctor was giving us all directions.

I'll try to explain what happened in the simplest of terms. When you have a patient who isn't pumping oxygenated blood and are in cardiac or respiratory arrest, you need to call the Code Blue, as noted.

Of course, before it's called there needs to be a quick assessment. So, someone checks for pulse. Someone checks to see if the patient is breathing. The big exception to all this is in the event the patient as a DNR order, which stands for do-not-resuscitate. Those are a whole different story.

DNR patients have legal orders stating they do not want to receive cardiopulmonary resuscitation (CPR) or advanced cardiac life support (ACLS).

I've encountered a lot of these in my career. And people generally do these for all different reasons. Sometimes it's religious. Sometimes it's just due to old age, and the patient is ready to go. Honestly, the why doesn't really matter. Your job is to just do the best job you can for them without breaking their wishes.

When you encounter a DNR who's in cardiac or respiratory arrest, you don't perform the same measures on them that you would normally do. As a matter of fact, you shouldn't call Code Blue to begin with.

In any event, our patient didn't have one, and, needless to say, things got chaotic quickly. Other professionals were rushing into the room. Various life-saving interventions were quickly initiated by the doctor.

The person who called the code in our case was the patient's nurse, and so she was the one who began CPR. I ended up assisting with the CPR until the decision was made to intubate the patient. You do this when you have to establish an effective airway.

All of our efforts proved ineffective, and sadly I must report that we lost the patient. I still recall walking out of the room with my head downplaying out the whole Code Blue in my head wondering if there was anything else I or we could have done.

Those are the kind of questions that haunt you like those red, fiery torches from my nightmare the previous nights.

I'm not symbologist, but in hindsight I've often tried to figure out what those torches meant or the piano keys getting pounded away to one of the most God-awful tunes I've ever heard in my life.

I can't say for sure, but I do sometimes think that the torches represented the lives of the patients I had lost. Except unlike the dream, once their torches went out, the patients were just gone and there was no bringing them back.

Now that's a haunting feeling. I wish I could share some happier moments from my time in New York, but I'd be lying if I didn't admit that the majority of my trip was a big whirlwind of pain, death, and misery.

Chapter 10

A Foreboding Feeling

No matter how hard I try I won't soon forget my third day at the hospital in the city or the young man that I met.

When I got to the hospital, I dawned my PPE and hit the ground running. The report from the other shift was distressing. Apparently, overnight they had lost several patients on this floor alone, a fact which startled me.

You know, as a medical pro you do occasionally have to deal with death. But dealing with death in such high numbers is like nothing I've ever saw. I was only on my third day at this point, and we'd already lost quite a few patients.

So, the Respiratory Department was jammed packed like normal. And I was making my rounds once again I caught my first alarm for the day. I hadn't been there maybe fifteen minutes tops, and it was already happening, and here I was still tired from tossing and turning the night before.

That's one of the big troubles with being on the frontline during a pandemic. It doesn't matter how tired you get, the virus just keeps coming at our necks like a relentless opponent. And some people seem to think that it only effects the elderly or people with pre-existing conditions, but that's simply untrue.

On this one such occasion, I had a noticeably young patient. This kid was only about 18-years-old, and he was scared out of his mind as you can imagine.

Now, normally kids that age will have parents close by, but, of course, since it was during this pandemic, he did not.

I quickly realized that the situation wasn't as dire at the moment as I had imagined, though.

The young man had just somehow managed to unplug one of the monitors on him. He wasn't on a vent yet – but he was in one of those precarious states where you felt like he could go on one at any moment.

"Do you play ball?" I asked noticing how athletic he looked. "You have to play ball, right?"

I just wanted to take his mind off everything that was happening.

His eyes were red and swollen, and he looked like he'd seen a ghost.

At first he didn't respond.

"You okay, my man?" I added checking the rest of his vitals. His oxygen wasn't great, but if it held firm he'd be okay.

He still didn't say anything. It could have been the medications, the illness, the whole situation. It's hard to say. But he was clearly worried and not wanting to talk with me or anyone.

I checked his vitals, looked him over, and started to move on. But something told me to stay just a little bit longer.

"Catch any good games lately?" I added.

His eyes darted up to mine, and I think I noticed a small grin etch itself across his face.

"So you do like sports?" I added, grinning.

He chuckled. That was the first smile or laugh I'd gotten from him, so I felt good about how things were going.

"You know what they used to tell me when I didn't want to talk?"

He shook his head no.

"They used to say, 'cat got your tongue.' I still don't know what the heck that means. Do you?" I asked.

He grinned.

"Nah," he said, shaking his head.

"So, you can talk!" I snapped. "The cat ain't got your tongue, huh?"

"Nah, it don't."

"It's nice to meet you young man. My name is James."

"What's yours?"

I knew his name from his chart, but I wanted him to talk. Maybe it would make him feel fetter.

"Walter."

"It's nice to meet you, Walter. I'm going to take really good care of you, okay?"

He nodded again.

"I bet you hate being asked do you play ball, right?" I added, repositioning his oxygen tubing.

"Yea, sometimes but I do play a little bit. Or, well, I used to before all this crap."

"Yea, I hear ya man. It's a crazy situation."

I continued to monitor his progress while he slowly opened up to me.

He was new to my floor and had Covid, and we were having trouble keeping his oxygen where we wanted to see it. So far, he was on the NRB mask, so the doctor hadn't switched him to a vent yet. Hopefully, that wouldn't be necessary because from what I could tell so far, once a patient goes on vent it's like their whole chances of success go down.

Honestly, some people even look at the vent like a death sentence, and while that's not completely true, it's certainly not something to be excited about. That's for sure.

"I hadn't talked to my mom since the other day," he added.

"Yea, this whole visitor policy thing is just terrible. I'm so sorry it has to be that way. It probably doesn't seem very fair."

"Can I ask you something, and I want you to be really honest with me?"

"Anything," I replied, letting him know he could talk to me if he wanted.

He looked at me and asked me if he was going to die. I don't know how many times I was asked this while in New York. Way too many to count.

What do you say to that?

Could you look at a teenage boy, one with the same skin tone as myself, and tell him the chances were fairly high he might not walk out of there alive?

Of course, you don't want to tell them anything like that. If you're anything like me, you want them to stay positive.

But the truth is, the case fatality rates were ridiculously high, especially early in the pandemic. They were even double digits in some countries like Italy. But you try not to think about stuff like that.

Besides, he wasn't on the vent yet, and hopefully we could keep it that way.

"You're ok man?" I told him. "I'm gonna try to do everything in my power to help you, too."

I've learned one indisputable fact in my life. There is a great deal of power in positive thought, which is why I always try to keep my patients happy and thinking about the future, even when their family isn't there to do that for them.

The truth was, in this kid's case, the virus may have started working it's way down the upper tract and into his lungs.

When it does that, the symptoms get far worse, which is why he was so short of breath, I figured.

I looked at his other vitals, too, and he was running a fever.

I checked his mask and made him perform some deep breathing techniques and asked him if everything was comfy or if I could get him anything.

"When can I see my mom?"

"I don't know. I'll try to find out, okay?"

I started to leave the room and paused.

"Hey, you know I've helped some of my other patients talk with their parents. One of them was able to connect on a FaceTime."

His eyes lit up.

I smiled.

"I'll see what I can do," I added and turned to walk away.

"James?" he asked.

I stopped.

"What's up man?"

"Thank you."

"You already know," I quipped and left the room.

. . .

That was not the extent of our conversation that day. Truth be told, I may have stayed in there a little bit longer than I should have, but all my other patients were stable at that moment.

I just felt a special kinship with the young man. He looked like me. He talked like me. He even acted like me a little bit.

Who am I kidding?

But at the end of the day, he just wanted to be with his mother, and if that wasn't possible, he wanted to talk with her.

So, I went about my rounds and then chatted with Jen. We became cool ever since our little incident. We had each other's backs. She really was a good nurse.

Sometimes things are so chaotic that you don't have time to stop and talk.

"I didn't think I was going to make it," she admitted.

"What do you mean? You're doing great, girl."

"Thanks to you."

"What the hell are you talking about?" I said, looking at the monitors, making sure my patients were okay.

"You helped me a lot on that first day. You've answered questions for me while you were here. I don't think I would have made it this far without you."

"Thank you. But don't thank me yet. Our adventure is far from over," I said, laughing.

"What time is it?" she asked.

"I think it's about time for night shift to roll in. We'll give this report and get home. How's that sound?"

"I'm with you on that," Jen said. "My feet are killing me."

After a few more odds and ends, I got ready to leave for the day not long after my brief conversation with Jen. She was a traveler like me, too, and I had met her on the first day I was there. I think she was more nervous than I was, but she is coming along, and I'm glad I was able to help her out.

After the report, I clocked out, and I stepped onto the elevator when a terrible feeling rushed over me.

Before the doors could close, I jumped out into the hallway, leaving everyone behind speechless.

"You okay?" Ydna yelled.

"I'm fine," I said. "Y'all go on without me. I forgot something."

What had I forgotten?

I hate to admit it.

But I had forgotten to help Walter. He wanted to call his mom, and the excitement of the day it had slipped my mind.

So, I ran to the secretary and talked to her, letting her know what was going on. She assured me that she would see to it that the young man got to call his mother.

Content that she would handle it I went home for the day. At the same time, I still had this foreboding feeling in the pit of my stomach.

Maybe it was all of the death and suffering. Maybe it was knowing that kid was down there wanting to talk to his damn mom and couldn't. I don't know. Maybe it was just everything piling up on me all at once.

I had only been there three days and was already wanting to leave. I was glad I was able to help Jen and the patients, but I was unsure how much longer I was going to make it myself.

Chapter 11

A Familiar Face

I had that awful feeling the whole way back to the hotel, but I was happy to see Sam's face when I walked inside.

He was standing at the desk and lit up when he saw me.

"How's your day?" he asked.

"Well, I'd like to say great, but it would be a lie."

"Oh, I'm sorry. Is there anything I can get for you?"

"Only if you have a cup of coffee or some liquor back there somewhere," I said, looking around. "I am exhausted, but I don't want to go to my room and pass out like I been doing."

"As a matter of fact," he said. "I just might be able to help you out. I'll be right back."

He disappeared somewhere, and I just stood there in the lobby wondering what the hell I was doing in that city. I was having nightmares. The job was busier than I ever imagined, and people were dying left and right.

Now, I had met this young man who was on his death's bed, and all he wanted to do was talk with his mother, and I somehow let that slip my mind.

That's not like me.

I'm glad I spoke with the secretary, though. Surely, I figured, she would handle it.

Things were taking a toll on me. There was no doubt.

When Sam returned with a fresh cup of hot, steaming coffee, I smiled one of those big, toothy smiles.

The little things in life, man!

We went and sat down across from one another in the lobby and started talking.

After a few minutes, I guess he could tell that I wasn't telling him everything, so he prodded some more. I'm more of a listener than a sharer. It's part of my empath nature.

"When you got here, I think you were ready to change the world," he said.

"And yet it's only been a few days, and I'm already on the verge of giving up. I just don't think I can do it. My gramps would be so pissed at me right now. He'd probably call me a quitter."

"Oh, I somehow doubt he would say that. You're not a quitter, James. You are a fighter or else you wouldn't be here right now. And you know what, I bet you your grandpa is looking out for you even if you don't yet realize it."

The thought of that honestly did make me feel better.

His words had a way of putting me at ease. Hell, I felt like I could tell him anything. Maybe I just hadn't been able to open up to anyone like that in a while, but it was sure as hell nice that he was willing to listen.

He also shared with me that he had taken my advice and called his own mother.

"That's what it's all about," I said. "'Family."

"You got that right."'

"Just keep that in mind when you're ready to give up. You got at least two people pulling for you, probably more."

"Who's that?"

"Me and your grandpa."

"That wasusp," I said. "'Thank you."

I finished sipping my coffee and then thanked him again for it – and the company.

Ever since this whole pandemic thing started, I've starved for human connections like a lot of you, I'm sure. Occasionally, though, there is a little beacon of light.

Sam was that light for me at that time.

At the same time, I just couldn't quite shake the memory of that young man in the hospital earlier. I really hoped that I would get to see him again soon, just as soon as my much-needed day off.

. . .

After about four days of working, I finally had a day off. I had taken part in so many Code Blues and other alarms that everything was starting to run together and blur.

I was also still a little bit haunted by the nightmare I had the other night, as well.

I could hear alarms going off and red and yellow lights flashing in my sleep. I could hear patients calling out to me. I could see patients falling over the side of their beds, ripping their tubes completely out.

Honestly, I probably couldn't tell you what all I did at work because it went by so fast. It was an amalgamation of emotion and caffeine – and when I set down to write this book I struggled to remember every detail I could. It wasn't easy.

I do remember death, though. It's not something you forget unless you proactively try to forget about it.

People were just dying all over the place as the trucks that were parked outside when I came the first day were replaced with new ones. The cycle repeats. It was just a sea of sick people in and out, and with no family in sight we were their only hope and only comfort.

Not to mention those God awful ventilators.

I guess you could say I was being hard on myself. I even started to question my skills as a Respiratory Therapist.

I doubted whether I was making a difference or not. I worried that I might get Covid, too, and end up on the same ventilators I was using on other people. I doubted the money was worth it any more. I felt like a dim light bulb with barely any shine left. I was just flickering ready to go out at any moment.

The mind can be your worst enemy if you allow it.

I wanted to quit. I even typed up my resignation. I made one copy for my agency and one for the hospital. I fell asleep with the intention of sending those letters out the next day and never step another foot inside that damn hospital again.

What changed?

My mindset.

Well, I had a strange dream later that night to be precise, and it was that dream that contributed to my shifting mindset. It's all quite hard to describe, but I'll do my best.

I was in a familiar place. This was nothing like the nightmare I had recently had.

My grandfather, who died when I was younger, came to visit me. And in the dream, I was sitting in his house where we used to live on Ashmont Street.

It felt so real. I think I was a child because he towered over me.

And there was that smiling face I often missed.

The smell of coffee and cigarettes singed my nostrils. The old man always had a fresh pot brewing, and he brought home the smell of cigarettes from the bar he owned and worked at.

I was in the living room watching television when he approached me.

"Looks like you're thinking about quitting," he said.

I stopped what I was watching briefly and stared up at the old man.

"I didn't know you were watching."

"I'm always watching."

My heart sank. I never wanted to do anything to let that man down. But it felt like he was scolding me. I was happy to see him, but it felt as if I was in trouble like when I was a kid, and he was mad at me.

He snatched the remote control I had in my hand and tossed against the wall. It smashed into a thousand little pieces.

I jumped up.

"What the hell did you do that for?"

"I think you know."

"What'd I do?"

He walked over to the old recliner he used to sit in and plopped down.

I paused for a minute as the anger started to slowly fade away. I missed the old guy. I couldn't stay mad at him for long.

"You are not quitter," he said. "You are smart, strong, and resourceful young man like I used to be," he proudly proclaimed.

I peered into his eyes as he spoke.

'You are right where you are supposed to be. And you have all the skills you need to succeed."

"Is this a dream?"

"Yup! You are definitely dreaming."

I chuckled.

I was simply happy to see the man.

He leaned back and expelled a huge cloud of smoke from the cigarette he had just lit.

"It is a dream," he added. "But the situation you're in is a test."

I nodded.

"You should always help as many people as you can and give comfort to those you can't because they appreciate it more than you may realize."

I watched in awe as he continued to speak.

"Don't be so hard on yourself," he said. "Your kind of a big baby like your grandmother was. She had a big heart full of empathy and compassion for others just like you. You probably got it from her."

"I miss her," I stated dropping my head down.

"You need to pep up you hear me?"

I nodded.

"You come from a strong family."

My eyes got really big.

"You'll be fine."

"I'm just tired."

Grandpa looked at me.

"You don't know tired," he added and took another long slow draw from the cigarette.

He let out a laugh, and I followed suit. He always knew exactly what to say. He wasn't a man of many words, but what he did say was always important.

I wish I could have kept him there with me just a little bit longer, but he eventually left. The last thing I recall was grandpa blowing out a large cloud of smoke as he faded into the background. Next thing I knew I was lying in bed.

Later that morning when I got up, I felt a new purpose, a renewed strength.

I had lost a few patients along the way. I had seen some things and been through some stuff.

But I wasn't a quitter.

After the dream – and wrestling with the decision to quit or not – I finally decided to keep pushing.

I wasn't going to quit on people who clearly needed me.

I felt like I had just experienced one of those scenes from the movies where a loved one comes to you and inspires you to keep going.

I know it's hard to believe, but that's what happened.

I genuinely believe my grandfather is my guardian angel. Whenever I want to give up on something, I am reminded of him.

It's his way of saying, "Hey, I'm here with you."

When I remember back, he used to push all of us grandkids to do better. Whether in school or life, he did not tolerate failure. And he reminded me in my dream to keep pushing forward no matter what.

I went for a walk earlier the next day and spent the rest day with Ydna. We became good friends and soaked up the fresh air at the park. It was peaceful because the streets were still empty and driving around was smooth and quick.

In my heart, I was ready to go back to work. I was ready to do what I could do to help.

No more slumping around. No more feeling defeated. I decided to change my mindset. And I grasped the fact I was in a major pandemic, and a lot of people were dying.

I had a renewed sense of confidence that I was going to help save as many people as possible, and I wanted to start with the young man I had met on my third day. For our purposes, we will call him Walter.

Chapter 12

Stormtroopers

After my much-needed day off, I practically ran into the hospital because I wanted to see Walter again and make sure he had spoken with his mom. I felt so terrible about not lining that up when he asked the first time, but it's so easy to lose track of things in all the chaos.

When I got to the floor I practically ran right passed Ydna and everyone else and went straight to his room and looked around.

There were four patients inside but not one of them was the young kid, Walter, whom I had just recently met.

He was gone.

I ran outside and down the hall to the front desk.

"Walter?" I said, practically shouting.

"Who?"

"The kid? The one in that room!" I said, pointing down the hall.

"209?"

"Um, yes, that's it. He was in 209. I checked on him yesterday. His name was Walter something. Where the hell is he?"

She looked around and then looked back at me confusedly.

"You didn't hear?"

"Hear what?"

"He's gone."

"Oh, he went home?"

"No, James. He didn't make it. I'm sorry. I thought you knew."

My heart sank all over again, and I felt the tears swell up inside. I left her standing there as I walked down the hall and then darted into the bathroom.

I don't know how I had made it that far without shedding a tear, but I wouldn't make it any longer.

I shed a few tears that day, which is totally against my normal persona. I'm this big, strong man. That's the me everyone sees – and knows. They probably think I'm completely impenetrable.

But some things just hit you right in the gut.

That one did.

Walter was gone.

I thought about him for a moment, the conversations we had together, and the fact that the last time we spoke he was needing to speak with his mother. That's all he really wanted, a familiar face amidst all the chaos, which is something I think we can all relate to.

I was devastated.

I don't know how long I was in there, but I ended up throwing some cold water on my face, quickly dried off, and fixed my PPE.

"Straighten your ass up, James," I said, looking into the mirror.

Just when I was feeling better after my dream last night and after a much-needed day off, I come in and get punched right in the stomach as soon as I get to work.

It's crazy.

But I know how this shit works. The focus of any hospital is simple. You must stabilize and treat the population of patients who arrive in the building.

Now, in the Respiratory Department we aren't seeing your standard accident victims or things like

109

that. We are making sure people can breathe (making sure that gaseous process I described earlier works likes it's supposed to).

You have to deliver timely, compassionate care in an uber-critical setting with often acute, life threatening illnesses like Covid.

The hospital there was filled with high tech equipment designed to treat a wide variety of maladies. But I also believe in what most doctors and nurses simply call bedside manner as well as the power of positive thought.

In other words, it's good to get the patient to be happy and thinking about positive things. But in the excitement of my day, I had somehow forgotten to help one of my patients connect with his mother, and that made me sick in hindsight.

I didn't ask how he died. I well knew. Covid does the same thing to all of its victims for the most part. I'll tell you how it tends to go down.

SARS-CoV2, which is the more official name for Covid, gets into your respiratory tract when you breathe in respiratory droplets that have the virus. That's the whole reason masks help, because we each have respiratory droplets in our breaths.

You can also get it from surfaces. In either case, the infection tends to begin in your nasal cavity. And it looks a little like one of those spiked medieval weapons shaped like a ball. The spikes consist of protein, and they are key to the viruses' being able to invade the cells in your respiratory tract.

They help the virus bind to ACE2, a protein on the surface of your cells; and it then tricks your cell into helping it get inside. It uses an enzyme named furin, which is present in the cells to break the protein spikes in half, allowing the spikes to guide the virus into your cells.

Once inside the cells, the virus hijacks your cells' machinery to make copies of itself. When they make enough, they start to invade additional cells lining your respiratory tract and begin to cause damage.

Like Walter's immune system, none of our immune systems have ever seen anything quite like SARS-CoV2 before.

His immune system would have scrambled to deal with the emergency with no real plan specific for the SARS-CoV2 strain. It cleverly dispatches it's evil little stormtroopers to the lining of your respiratory tract, making it a veritable battleground for your soul.

If everything remains in your upper respiratory tract (above your trachea), your immune system may be capable of winning the war. That's true for a lot of people. It wasn't true for Walter and countless others like him.

The problem for him was that the infection proceeded down his respiratory tract and into his respiratory tree and lungs. That's why he was short of breath when we spoke.

Other symptoms he had were chest pain and tightness, a deep cough, and sheer and utter difficulty breathing except for that NRB mask.

Now, at the end of the respiratory tract are these balloon-like structures called alveoli, which may sound like an Italian pasta dish but instead are membranous structures that fill with the air you inhale.

The alveoli are intertwined with a network of blood vessels that bring blood from the rest of the body that is low in oxygen and high in carbon dioxide (which is a waste product of metabolism).

These alveoli serve as swaps where oxygen from the air you breathed is exchanged with the carbon dioxide in your blood. The carbon dioxide goes into the alveoli, where it's exhaled up through the respiratory tract and out the nose and mouth.

The blood that's infused with oxygen travels to the rest of the body to provide fuel for all your cells to live.

Does that make sense? That's why the lungs are so important. When the alveoli don't work right, the body gets starved of oxygen and is unable to get rid of the carbon dioxide. Things go downhill after that happens. This was no doubt the case with my friend.

If you didn't know, pneumonia is when your alveoli become inflamed and fill up with fluid, pus, and other gunk (i.e., cells and other stuff). This can happen in one or both the lungs, and developing a pneumonia is when the infection really gets serious.

It wasn't just with Walter. I just kept seeing this play out over and over throughout all my weeks in New York.

Of course, I didn't stay hidden away crying in the bathroom forever. Hardly. That's just not me. It's not who I am. But that one did hurt.

At the same time, I knew I had to pull myself up and keep pushing.

In this profession, there are literally thousands of Walters. And sometimes you lose some of them. You do all you can, and sometimes it doesn't work out.

So, I ended up bursting back out of the bathroom a few minutes later. I came into the hall with my head held high determined to check on the rest of my patients.

"You okay?" Jen asked.

"Never better," I quipped, lying. "How's that patient in 220?" I asked.

We were quickly back to work. I guess you could say were stormtroopers. The virus was treating these folks' bodies like a battleground. And it was time to tighten up.

. . .

And I'm glad I did. Later on in our shift, I had a young Latino patient, Manuel, who had survived Covid remarkably well so far. I had physician's orders to go and try and take him off the vent to see how he would do without it.

He did survive, but unfortunately, he ended up with a tracheostomy and was still on the vent. A tracheostomy provides direct access to your lungs through a hole in your windpipe or trachea.

We often trach patients who still need help breathing. Tracheostomies allow us to take out the breathing tube that goes through the mouth or nose and into the lungs. By doing this, we can work on getting patients completely off ventilators and back to normal.

I had walked into the patient's room, which was the farthest away from the main nursing station. The patient was the only one in there, and he was staring at the ceiling. He must have tried to grab an ice cup because he had ice spilled all over him.

I introduced myself as I cleaned up all the spilled ice. He just stared at me as I spoke. I explained to him that I was there to take him off the machine and see how he did on his own. I told him that I would be there the entire time to make sure he was ok.

He tried to mouth something to me. Patients with trachs may not be able to speak on the vent, but most of the time, I can read lips.

He was mouthing so fast I couldn't make out the words. I told him I was going to go grab a paper and pencil, so he could write.

After I had told him that, he grabbed me, and I read his lips, "Please don't leave."

He said it clear as day.

You could see the fear and anxiety in his eyes. But I stressed to him that I would be right back.

I had quickly grabbed a pen and paper from the secretary and gave it to my patient to write. He struggled to write at first because he was so weak.

He eventually jotted down, "You see me?"

I told him of course and that he was not, in fact, invisible, the thought of which still makes me smile.

He then jotted that the words, "People just walk by. I'm scared."

My face dropped.

My heart ached for him. He was right.

It's so easy to think about things through the eyes of the doctors, nurses, RTs, and other medical professionals. I get that. And that's a big part of what this story is all about, I presume.

But what happens when you turn the attention on the patient?

They see all of us like hordes of cattle, I imagine. We're coming in and out and there's hardly any real compassion, I would add.

It comes with the job. For one, you can't get tied down to just one patient when so many others need you. And you can't let your emotions get the best of you either. Then you're doing a disservice to the people you are bound to help.

114

There's a fine line between just making your rounds and keeping your mind as clear as possible from all the emotions that inevitably arise and having good bed side manner, which is something you've heard me address throughout this tale.

I've also found it helpful to let the patients know what's going on. So, I paused what I was doing and sat him up and explained to him his present condition and what we were trying to do to help him.

Now, this particular patient had been with the hospital since before I got there. So, he had already come so far. He was one of the bright spots during my trip to New York. And I reminded him that he'd be at home in no time.

As I left his room that day his eyes were tearing up, but I think he recognized how far he had come. Manuel was a fighter.

Chapter 13

The Who, What, and Why

The rest of the week went off without a hitch, and I can honestly say that I'm thankful I had my guardian angel with me, my grandpa. Plus, I would still sometimes think about Walter and other patients I had, some of whom I lost, but in a weird way it gave me strength.

If you recall Manuel, he kept making improvements the whole time I was there. And the promise I made him that he'd be going home soon was looking more and more likely that it would be true.

One day, I came into his room and he was just waking up. I checked his vitals, and everything looked fine.

"Have you gotten to speak with your family yet, Manuel?"

He nodded.

When I mentioned his family, he lost it. Tears came down his face like a rushing waterfall. I pulled up a chair, sat in it, and told him to look at me because he was hysterical at that point.

I told him to believe in himself and to see that he was still there. A lot of times patients get discouraged and forget about the progress that they've made. People want to expedite recovery.

I gave him some tissues and told him to wipe his tears because he had a job to do. I told him his job was to get better. I told him he needed to treat his recovery like a job. Punch the clock, put in the work, and then go home.

He started to cheer up.

Sometimes you just must have real conversations with patients and snap them out of the sunken place they're in. You'd be surprised how much a positive spirit can help physically, too.

That gentleman got my message loud and clear. He perked up. For the first time since I met him, he had a smile on his face. I explained to him that we were going to be taking him off the ventilator and put some oxygen on him and see if he was ready.

I let him know it would feel a little bit weird at first. He had been on the vent for a month at that point according to my records. That's a very long time to have something help you breathe, and if you recall from earlier, I was talking about how precarious the situation is once someone goes on a vent. Their chances of survival tend to go down considerably.

Once I had taken him off the machine and placed him on oxygen, he did fine, though, and I was so excited to see that.

As a matter of fact, he actually did more than fine. Manuel did very well especially for someone who had been on the vent. You could see that he was a little anxious, but that is normal for most patients when they first come off the ventilator. They almost forget that they are capable of breathing on their own.

I checked his vitals again. His heart rate was still normal, and with the little extra oxygen I gave him his body was still at 100%. I turned the monitor to him and showed him his numbers. By doing that, it looked like I eased some of his anxiety.

At that point, I told him I had to go. I still had a full assignment that I had to get to, but I had to make sure this guy did not lose his mind while he was in the hospital. And he was doing well enough for him to leave soon.

I called his nurse into the room and explained what I had just done. We planned to keep him off the ventilator for at least four hours. If he did good with the four hours, then we would extend it four more and reassess from there.

I had to do a few more things for him before I left. And I told him to press the red button if he felt like he was having trouble breathing or if he needed anything. The nurse also got him an iPad so he could FaceTime his family.

As I walked out of the room, I heard what sounded like a female voice answer the FaceTime and scream when she saw him. Now, that was the first good scream I had heard lately.

And, in case you were wondering, Manuel not only got to speak with his family that day, he got to leave the hospital within about two weeks of coming off the vent.

I didn't get to see the reunion with his family when he walked out, but you don't have to have much of an imagination to know that it probably went well.

Something about his story gave me strength, too. I ended up using that strength and the support of my guardian angel to help take care of a lot of patients on ventilators.

As stated before, a lot of it was a blur. It was incredibly difficult trying to remember each and every small detail, but I did my best. I also changed the names of some of the patients for obvious reasons. There's HIPAA to take into consideration, plus it's just the right thing to do.

All told, the next few weeks went by pretty fast and every day was hectic and exhausting. Patients became room numbers and vent numbers. It was almost impossible to try and remember all the names. But certain ones stood out to me the most, I guess you could say.

You can't forget all the Manuel's and Walters of the world. Some of them got to go on living – and we are unsure as of yet what all the long-lasting effects of the virus entail. But some of them did not get to live and died well before they should have.

There was this seemingly endless sea of black and brown bodies on those damn vents, and that still bothers me to this day. Anyone can get Covid. Don't get me wrong, but it seems to affect Latinos and African Americans the hardest.

Each room I walked in was a similar scene, mostly black and brown people suffering, crying out for family.

I would sometimes freeze momentarily when I entered a room, especially in those early days of the trip. I was in total disbelief. Covid is devouring all races, but it apparently had a taste for us folks with darker skin tones for some reason.

I've often reflected on exactly why that is, but, again, I think that's the subject for someone else's book.

As if most of these patients didn't already face hardships in life because of their skin tone, now a virus was singling them out. It wasn't fair. This fueled my desire to help them even more, though.

Someone had to give them a chance. I could have been one of those patients in a bed. It could have been me clinging to life while my body craved more and more oxygen to feed its dying cells.

. . .

I noted that my days started to blur and that I couldn't remember all the patients. Soon patients became numbers and rooms. But that's not the entire story. There was Walter and Manuel and a few others that seemed to stand out the most.

In one such instance, the physicians said they were having a hard time getting the patient off a vent. He was a young guy. We'll call him Jose.

He had to be about twenty-one and Latin-American. They said he kept failing his spontaneous breathing trial (SBT).

For perspective, an SBT allows doctors to see if a patient can breathe on their own while on the ventilator. Usually, to pass an SBT, you must be stable for the duration of it. This could be anywhere from 30 minutes to an hour. And it lets us know how the patient will do if we take them off the machine.

I pulled up his chart to see what some reasons could be why he was failing his trial. According to the chart, every time he failed, it was due to his vitals becoming unstable. His heart rate would go up, and his respiratory rate would go up, as well. Every time he failed; it would ultimately extend his time on the ventilator.

After I had all the information I needed, I touched base with the nurse to see if she had cut off his sedation. The sedation keeps the patient sleepy and comfortable while on the machine. We needed him awake and alert for the trial. She said the sedation had been off for about an hour, and I was all set to start the trial.

When I laid eyes on him, I noticed he was staring at the ceiling with his eyes racing back and forth. The first thing I did was to raise his bed up so that he was sitting up comfortably.

Everyone was always so busy and forgot the small things that make a big difference when it came to patient comfort. The first thing is to sit them up, so they are not counting ceiling tiles all day.

The second thing was to be there when they started waking up off sedation and explain what was happening. A lot of patients start to wake up from sedation and are confused and scared. They want to know what's going on.

Imagine waking up on a breathing machine alone in a room by yourself. Imagine not facing the door. You don't see what's going on, but you can hear everything. You hear people talking in a medical language that you don't understand. You hear people walking in and out of other room tending to patients.

So, I introduced myself to the young gentleman. I told him I was there to help get the breathing tube out. I told him about the SBT, and that if he passed, we could remove the tube.

Jose's eyes were fixed on me (I changed his name as I did with others). I know he had a lot of questions and was frustrated that he could not ask them because of the tube.

I explained to him that for the trial, he would still be on the machine, but it wouldn't be helping him. I explained he would be doing all the work on his own, as if the machine was not there.

The trial started, and instantly, he was breathing well on his own. I stayed right by his side to monitor him and his vitals.

After ten minutes went by, I told him I was going to find his doctors to let them know that he was doing good and that the tube was most likely going to come out. He was still fixed on me. I told him he was doing so well and that the trial would last a little bit longer. I could not have emphasized enough how well he was doing. I wanted him to feel confident about his breathing.

When I got to the desk and spoke with the doctors, the nurse called and said his heart rate had increased dramatically. An unstable or increased heart rate is grounds to fail someone on an SBT. The doctor had heard the nurse and told me to cancel the trial and that we would try again tomorrow.

I told the doctor that I thought it was anxiety and that the patient was scared to be alone. I asked him to go in the room with me. I wanted him to see the patient for himself. I wanted to see how fast the young man's heart rate would go back to normal once someone was in the room with him.

When we got to the room and started to speak to the patient, his heart rate quickly returned to normal. It took him maybe thirty seconds to settle down completely. He was scared, anxious, and didn't want to be alone.

After the doctor saw the patient calm, he looked at me and said, "Go ahead and extubate."

That is the fancy medical word for "Pull the tube." All it took was for someone to take a little extra time to even notice that patient was failing because of anxiety. He could have been off this machine days ago.

When I finally pulled the tube out, the patient took the biggest breath of air he could. It was like he just swam to the surface of the water after a twenty-foot plunge and took in the most amount of air he could.

Then he let it out and just looked so grateful and thankful. My heart did about six back flips. You could see the relief on the patient's face. You could see the joy in his eyes. He probably didn't even think he was going to make it.

Sometimes no matter how busy you are, you must slow down. Do not miss the little things. In our haste, we tend to overlook key details.

Sometimes, while we're working, our bodies are moving, but we are not really processing what is happening. It's like autopilot. If there is one thing that a patient doesn't need, it's an autopilot employee. When you feel you're in autopilot, please stop and remember the who, what, and why.

The who are all the Walter's, Manuel's, and Jose's who needed us. The what is this sick medieval looking virus called SARS-CoV2 or Covid-19 or coronavirus. It is incredibly effective as a killing machine and wages war below the upper tract. And the why is the easiest of all …

It's because we care.

Chapter 14

An Invitation

There was so much more stuff that I witnessed while working in a New York City hospital. Horrible things. Unspeakable things. A lot of patients died from Covid, but a lot of them died from other things, as well. I could not have possibly shared all of their stories, but as noted, a few of them tended to stand out to me more than others.

There was Walter, God rest his soul. He lost his battle with Covid while praying to see his mom's face again. There was Jose and Manuel who survived this terrible battle with the disease despite it having lurched below their upper tracts and causing pneumonia. They were vented, but unlike some of the others, they ended up surviving.

Each of these patients represented someone's family member. It was the son or daughter. It was the cousin or niece or nephew. It was someone's uncle or aunt or grandparent.

Each one had a name. Each one had a purpose. And that purpose was cut short right there on the frontlines of this war with coronavirus.

What's worse, most of these patients never got to see their loved ones when they passed. They never got to take that job or date that person they admired.

Some probably even had petty, unresolved arguments lingering with friends, arguments that seem minuscule in retrospect.

I'm sure they had planned vacations, weddings, and birthday parties to attend. They had kids who will now grow up parentless.

They had parents who now must bury their children. The saddest part of all was the fact that most of the patients who died did not get to say their goodbyes either and that still hurts me.

So, why do I say all of this?

I certainly don't mean to be so negative. Like Jose and Manuel, there were some bright spots along the way, thank God, or I think I would have never made it.

Jose and Manuel gave me hope when I had so very little. Couple that with my own little guardian angel at my side the whole time, and I would find an extra gear that I never knew I had.

And despite all of the losses I witnessed, it did get better, too. By better, I mean fewer people were being admitted into the ICU with this terrible virus from the moment I got there until I left. Fewer people were coming through the ER. Fewer people were on our floor. And thank God, fewer people had to be vented.

The quarantine seemed to have really slowed the spread of the virus, especially in New York, because things had gotten bad there for a while.

It went from extremely busy and chaotic to slow and almost empty in a matter of weeks, which is cause to celebrate.

Covid came in like riptide, sucked up an overwhelming amount of people, and then started to slowly dissipate.

The mood in the city lifted as the weather got better, as well. People started coming out of their homes and going to parks. Outdoor activities spiked because you could maintain a safer distance from people.

The city had plans to start reopening in phases. People were eager to get back to their businesses. I was eager to go home and take a break. And I didn't want to see another ventilator for a while.

I remember one of my last days there I finally got to visit Central Park. During the pandemic, I worked so many hours that I didn't have much time for myself. And when I did have a day off I was so tired that I didn't really feel like doing much.

But as things started to slowly dissipate, I finally took the time to take in a few of the sites of the city. I've always loved the Big Apple. And I will never forget my time there during the pandemic.

I learned a lot during my trip. I learned that I'm tougher than I once thought I was. I learned there are great people out there like Sam, Ydna, Jen, Jose, and countless others.

I learned that life is too short, and we should really enjoy the time we have. We can all be gone in a blink of an eye.

I invite you to live without regret and do what you love. Do whatever makes you happy.

If I had a choice to do this all over again, I'm not sure that I would. No one should have to go through that. I'm glad it's in the history books, so maybe future generations can avoid this sort of thing from happening again.

To all the families who lost a loved one due to this virus, my heart breaks for you.

They say time heals all wounds, and I truly believe it helps. But the pain will carry on for some time.

In the meantime, please accept this invitation to celebrate your lost family members. Share their positive stories. Remember all the good times. And, lastly, don't be so hard on yourself either. Your loved ones know you loved them with all of your heart.

So, be kind to yourself and allow yourself to grieve properly.

Lastly, if you'd like some additional information on the virus check out the appendix. Since I began writing this book, there were some alarming statistics coming out about ventilators, much of which I witnessed myself.

Peace to you all!

Appendix

Additional Resources

In the days and weeks since I wrote this manuscript, the virus has continued to rage on throughout the United States. We now have over 6 million cases and 185,000 Covid deaths as of the end of August. You've also probably read or heard a lot about ventilators, and so I wanted to include some info on those here, as the use of them are very much a part of my job.

A lot of these things I learned on my own, but I will say there was a major study that examined outcomes for more than 2,600 patients found an extraordinarily high death rate of 88% among Covid-19 patients in New York City who had to be placed on mechanical devices to help them breathe.[1] Some of those 2,600 patients I worked on myself as a Respiratory Therapist, so I can speak to the accuracy of those claims.

The study was published in the *Journal of the American Medical Association*, which is one of the largest reviews published to date on Covid-19 patients hospitalized in this country.

From what I understand, the researchers examined outcomes for Covid-19 patients who were admitted between March 1 and April 4 to 12 hospitals in New York City and Long Island that are part of the Northwell Health system.[2]

Overall, the researchers reported that 553 patients died which is 21%. But among the 12% of very sick patients that needed ventilators to help them breathe, the death rate rose to an astounding 88%.

The rate was particularly awful for patients over the age of 65 who had to be placed on a machine. Only 3% of those patients survived per the results of that same study. And, the study found, that men had a higher mortality rate than women.

The authors of the study wrote, "The findings of high mortality rates among ventilated patients are similar to smaller case series reports of critically ill patients in the US."[3]

With no drugs that are proven, ventilators are one of the go-to options for ICUs and critical care units in dealing with severe cases of Covid-19 pneumonia.

However, there are growing reports that very few patients who get on the machine are able to get off of it, which I can also say is true. As a result, some doctors question the use in Covid-19 patients and have been trying to find methods for keeping their patients off them if possible.

At the same time, I fear that the mortality rate in the study may not represent the ultimate picture that may emerge. For one, the study only included patients for whom a definite outcome is already known, meaning those who died or were discharged. It did not, for example, include patients still being treated, which would likely lessen the death rates. For more on the study, refer to the following endnotes.

Endnotes

[1]https://jamanetwork.com/journals/jama/fullarticl
e/2765184
[22]https://www.bloomberg.com/profile/company/16
47803D:US
[3]https://www.bloomberg.com/news/articles/2020-
04-22/almost-9-in-10-covid-19-patients-on-
ventilators-died-in-study